D1360515

Praise for Health Is Wealth

"takes a natural, commonsense approach"

"The answers to attaining and maintaining great health and longevity are found in Dr. Senne's book *Health Is Wealth*, which takes a natural, commonsense approach to physical, mental, emotional, social, and spiritual health. This book has made an incredible difference in my life and I highly recommend it to all those seeking better health."

DR. MERRIL BERG, D.ED., M.ED.
President Emeritus, Lake Region State College

"conversational . . . yet very informative."

"Readers will find *Health Is Wealth* to be an enjoyable book and one that is very applicable for their health and well-being. Dr. Senne presents the book in a conversational, and yet very informative manner that the reader will appreciate."

GOVERNOR ARTHUR A. LINK
Former Governor of North Dakota

"a Bible on Health"

"Finally, a book has been written encompassing the physical, mental, spiritual, emotional, and social dimensions pertaining to our health. Dr. Senne presents *Health Is Wealth* in a passionate and very informative manner that invites the reader to take a journey on the road to excellent health by implementing the easy-to-follow recommendations outlined in his book. *Health Is Wealth*, simply put, is a Bible on Health."

DR. MARCOS RAMOS
Professor, Florida Center for Theological Studies

HEALTH IS
WEALTH

THE PATH TO ENRICHING
YOUR LIFE & YOUR HEALTH

DR. SCOTT C. SENNE

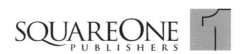

SQUAREONE
PUBLISHERS

The information and advice contained in this book are based upon the research and the personal and professional experiences of the author. They are not intended as a substitute for consulting with a health care professional. The publisher and author are not responsible for any adverse effects or consequences resulting from the use of any of the suggestions, preparations, or procedures discussed in this book. All matters pertaining to your physical health should be supervised by a health care professional. It is a sign of wisdom, not cowardice, to seek a second or third opinion.

COVER DESIGNER: Jeannie Tudor
FRONT COVER PHOTOS: Getty Images, Inc.
BACK COVER PHOTO: Dave Parmelee
IN-HOUSE EDITOR: Joanne Abrams
TYPESETTER: Gary A. Rosenberg

Square One Publishers
115 Herricks Road
Garden City Park, NY 11040
(516) 535-2010 • (877) 900-BOOK
www.squareonepublishers.com

Library of Congress Cataloging-in-Publication Data

Senne, Scott C.
  Health is wealth : the path to enriching your life & your health /
Scott C. Senne.
     p. cm.
  Includes bibliographical references and index.
  ISBN 978-0-7570-0356-1 (pbk.)
  1. Health. 2. Naturopathy. I. Title.
  RA776.S457 2010
  613--dc22

                                                              2010010244

Printed in Canada

10   9   8   7   6   5   4   3   2   1

Contents

This book is dedicated to my family,
in particular my wife, Linda;
my daughter, Sommer Lynn; my son, Shiloh Ray;
my mother, Phyllis Ratcliffe; my sister in-law, Jean Wald;
and my dear friend Gloria Mickelson.

It is also dedicated to the many people
I was honored to have as patients and to the many
who have attended my speaking engagements.

A Word About Gender

In an effort to avoid awkward phrasing within sentences, it is our publishing style to alternate the use of male and female pronouns according to chapter. Therefore, when referring to a "third-person" adult, child, healthcare provider, or caregiver, odd-numbered chapters will use female pronouns, while even-numbered chapters will use male, to give acknowledgment to people of both genders.

Acknowledgments

Linda: I would like to thank you for fourteen years of marriage. You are a wonderful wife and mother to our two children. You stood beside me during all my years of undergraduate and graduate college, and throughout all the phases of my professional healthcare career. You helped me to become a better doctor, husband, and father, and I am eternally grateful that God has blessed me with you as my wife.

Sommer: It has been a privilege to be your father for these past ten years. You are a beautiful young lady both inside and out. I have matured as a man watching you grow, and helping you to uncover all the talents and abilities that God has given you. You have helped me uncover hidden talents and abilities that God has given me that I was unaware I had. The day you were born brought a powerful change in my life. You are my angel. Thank you for being such a bright light in my life.

Shiloh: You are only eleven months old and you are truly a gift from God, as this is what your name means. I am looking forward to seeing the kind of man that God will have you become. You are a strong little boy both mentally and physically, and I anticipate with great pleasure the guiding and directing that I trust God will give me in helping to shape your life. You have taught me how to look deep inside myself. You are my little man and a joy to hold next to my heart. You make me smile and laugh and appreciate God's wonderful creation.

Judy Reveal: Thank you, Judy, for editing *Health Is Wealth*. I appreciate your professionalism and your commitment to excellence. It has been a real pleasure working with you. I consider you not only a wonderful editor but a friend as well.

Rich Mintzer: Thank you for your guidance, intuitiveness, and recommendations in the second editing of *Health Is Wealth*. Your experience and knowledge in presenting material was very much appreciated. It has been a joy and honor to work with you.

Joanne Abrams: I extend to you a very special thank-you for bringing the whole book together. Your editorial professionalism and attention to detail made the book come into focus. It has been a joy to work with you.

Deb Hoeffner: Thank you, Deb, for the artwork that you provided at the end of each chapter. The footprints beautifully capture the theme of the book as readers embark upon their personal journeys to health and wellness.

Les Stobbe: I would like to send a thank-you for your belief and faith in the project.

Rudy Shur: I would like to thank you for accepting this project. Your knowledge, integrity, sincerity, and honesty are like a beacon of light in the publishing world. I am honored that *Health Is Wealth* is part of the Square One team of books.

Preface

There I sat in the doctor's office. It was the fall of 1980 and oh, did my foot hurt! For the past six months, I had been preparing for the state championship in cross-country racing. I thought about this autumn race every morning as I laced up my shoes and headed out the door for my early morning run. I wanted to be state champion! I was excited because I was actually ranked as a favorite to finish in first place. Some very good runners were going to be in the race, but I had just as good a chance of winning as they did, for I had beaten each of them at one time or another during that season or the previous one.

I wasn't some person just out for glory; running was something that came very naturally to me and something that I loved. I had tried out for the junior high cross-country team and had found immediate success. I suppose it is only natural to enjoy something that you're good at, and I definitely became good at running. I enjoyed the sense of freedom it afforded me. I enjoyed running in all kinds of weather, at any time of the year. Best of all, I didn't have to rely on anyone else for my success or failure in the sport. It was up to me to put in the training—or to stay in my nice, warm bed.

So there I was at the doctor's office, dutifully waiting my turn. The doctor finally appeared long after the scheduled time, and I was given a curt hello and asked what I wanted. I told the doctor that my foot hurt and asked if he could please take a look at it. The doctor looked at me as if I was an unwelcome intrusion into his day. With no apologies or acknowledgment of the fact that he was behind schedule, he hurriedly told me to take off my shoe. I asked the doctor why my foot hurt, when it would get better, how I could prevent the pain from occurring again, and most of all, how he could help me. After all, I had a lot riding on what he had to say. With one glance at my foot, the doctor said, "Take these pills!"

"Take these pills!" I thought. How is this pill going to go all the way down to my foot and help it? I asked the doctor what my diagnosis was and he gave me a long medical answer that I didn't understand. He made no attempt to help me grasp the problem. I later came to realize that his diagnosis was some fancy word that simply meant "sore foot." I wanted answers, but what I got was a brush-off.

That "doctor's" visit certainly made a lifelong impression on me. That was the day that my journey into healthcare began, and it was in that office that I decided to one day become a doctor. I would help my patients understand what their diagnosis was, how they had developed their problem in the first place, what could be done to make them feel better, and how they could prevent the problem from occurring in the future. I was going to give my patients answers. I would be their doctor, friend, and healthcare teammate. They wouldn't hear from me, "Take two aspirin and call me in the morning!" Or, as in my case, "Don't call me in the morning."

I wanted to learn everything I could about the body. I wanted to help as many people with their various health conditions as I could. I went on to college to complete my bachelor's degree, and then to graduate school, where I obtained my doctorate. I never forgot my dream of helping patients. As for the cross-country meet, unfortunately, my foot did not heal in time.

Receiving my doctorate was only the first step in learning to help people improve and regain their health. My education taught me a great deal about the body, but it was through seeing patients that I really learned how to take care of people. I recognized that patients are not just a sum of their parts. Each patient is a whole, unique person, and that unique individual—not just his symptoms—needs to be treated with care and respect.

As a result of my approach, my healthcare center attracted patients throughout the Midwest. I routinely saw people who had driven several hundred miles to reach my clinic. I was honored not only to treat them as patients, but also to call them my friends and become teammates with them in their healthcare. My dream of helping people had come true.

After practicing for ten years, I became a healthcare consultant. It was hard to step down from caring for patients on a daily basis, but I felt that if I could work with other doctors and assist them with their practices, I could, in effect, treat even more people. I also established a healthcare lecture series for the public. The response to this series proved to be overwhelming, and made me aware of how many people long for a commonsense, holistic approach to good health. It was this awareness that spurred me on to write this book so that people everywhere could learn how to improve their well-being not only on a physical level, but also mentally, emotionally, socially, and spiritually. It is my hope that this book will serve as a guide and companion as you work toward greater health and happiness for yourself and your family.

Dr. Scott C. Senne

Foreword

n today's world of processed foods, polluted air, and toxic water, you need a guide to lead you along the road to good health. *Health Is Wealth* takes you on a journey designed to enhance your physical, mental, spiritual, emotional, and social health and well-being. I have been using many of principles discussed in this book in my own treatment center over the years, and have found them to be very effective in helping my patients. I am confident that you can improve your own health by implementing the advice offered in these pages.

The information in *Health Is Wealth* is presented in an easy-to-read format with plenty of case histories that demonstrate how Dr. Senne's suggestions can be incorporated into your daily routine. Rather than focusing on symptoms, *Health Is Wealth* takes a whole body approach to healthcare. This means that the changes you make will not just alleviate your symptoms, but also improve your overall well-being as well as your outlook on life.

Health Is Wealth is designed as a step-by-step journey, with each chapter bringing you one step closer to attaining and maintaining good health. As you move through the book and implement Dr. Senne's advice, you will notice a continual improvement in your well-being. Yet Dr. Senne is realistic in his approach; he knows that you may not implement every single suggestion presented in the book. You can choose and benefit from the lifestyle changes that make sense to you. And you can rest assured that Dr. Senne's suggestions are backed by thorough research and years of clinical experience.

Health Is Wealth is not about depriving yourself of the things you really want. It is about replacing harmful habits with healthful habits. This makes Dr. Senne's suggestions easy to follow. You will learn that you don't have to turn your life upside down to enhance your health.

Traveling the road to wellness is a joyful experience, as each step of the journey improves your life in so many ways. This book leads you along this path with Dr. Senne by your side, offering you encouragement and support. May God bless and enrich your well-being as you read *Health Is Wealth*.

Dr. Gregory L. Jantz, PhD, CEDS
Founder of The Center: A Place of Hope
Best-selling author of *The Body God Designed*

Introduction

There are a lot of diet, health, and exercise books on the market today. Many promise to provide a quick cure if you use a particular piece of exercise equipment, take a new pill, apply the latest cream, or follow a special diet.

Authors of health books often admonish their readers for not knowing which way to turn, or blame drug companies and doctors for being ill-informed or for simply turning a blind eye to proper healthcare. This book is not about pointing fingers or making any individual or group feel bad. Instead, it is designed to help you understand why you become sick and what you can do to attain, regain, and maintain excellent health the natural way. This is not an arduous book to get through, and you won't need to feverishly take notes and go through a box of highlighters. I wrote this book as if I were talking to my patients. I would like you to view me as a friend, doctor, and teammate regarding your healthcare issues. I will take this journey with you down the road of health, and if you follow my easy-to-implement suggestions along the way, you will achieve excellent health by the end of the journey.

How many people actually wake up every day and say "I feel great"? Such people are ready to take on each day with a fresh enthusiasm. They are on no medications and they look as good as they feel. They are vibrant most days of the year, and they may even seem to be getting younger instead of older. Well, there are a lot of people who do *not* fall into this category! This is unfortunate, because so many more people could wake up saying, "I feel great!" You have the power to choose the type of person you become.

Our bodies are efficient machines, capable of performing great feats of strength and endurance when called upon. In most cases, though, modern life does not require us to perform feats of strength and endurance for our survival. Instead, each day, we are required to manage an intricate balancing of jobs, family, and friends that can leave us feeling stressed-out. Unlike a real machine, however, the human body does have the ability to repair and heal itself. Did you know that all of the cells in the body, except the nerve cells, actually reproduce throughout the course of a day, week, month, and year? We get a new body every year! Doesn't it make sense to take care of ourselves as well as we possibly can? I want my new cells to be strong and sound. I want my new body to be even healthier than my previous body!

Throughout this book, I share with you my recommendations for attaining and maintaining excellent health the natural way while getting to the cause of sickness, disease, and degenerative conditions. Over the years, I have offered these recommendations to my family, to a multitude of patients, to audience members, and to healthcare professionals, and have found that, when followed, my guidelines produce great results. Case studies, provided throughout the book, show how others have dramatically improved their health by making the simple changes I suggest.

Each chapter of this book focuses on a different topic, from healthy water to a beneficial home environment. In the following pages, I would like to touch upon some of the most important principles you'll find in *Health Is Wealth*.

FUELING THE BODY

One of my most important recommendations is to obtain good nutrition as a means of improving your body's performance. It is a fact that most people put more thought into their car's performance than their own performance. They get regular oil changes, radiator flushes, tire rotations, and air pressure checks. They choose the most appropriate form of fuel for their car, but they don't pay much attention to the fuel they put in their own body, nor do they know about the body flushes that can help maintain optimum health.

Most people don't think too much about their health until they lose it, and then they simply look for a way to "fix" it. This usually involves taking pills, but while pills may hide the symptoms of pain or dysfunction, they rarely correct the root cause. I like to compare taking a pill to using a bucket to prevent a leak in the ceiling from flooding the house. If you repaired the crack in the ceiling, you wouldn't have to worry about emptying buckets of water. Similarly, if you addressed the cause of your health disorder, you wouldn't have to worry about taking pills and potentially setting your body up for more serious health problems down the road.

Many times, symptoms disappear as a result of taking a pill, but that does not mean the problem is fixed. It simply means that your body has, for the time being, stopped trying to get your attention through gentle nudging. Sooner or later, if the cause of the problem is not addressed, your body will shout at you, and at that point, your disorder will most likely be much more difficult to correct. The old adage, "An ounce of prevention is worth a pound of cure," is never more appropriate than when discussing your health. A small investment in a healthy lifestyle now—including the best possible nutrition—will pay big dividends as you go through life.

GETTING TO THE ROOT OF THE PROBLEM

When I graduated from school, I thought I knew a lot about helping patients. Boy, was I in for a shock! When I first started practicing, I would give my patients a form to fill out. To complete the form, patients had to check the box next to every part of their body that gave them pain, and describe the type and severity of the pain and how it negatively affected their lives. The form covered everything, including the nervous (nerves, brain, and spinal cord), circulatory (arteries, veins, and capillaries), cardiovascular (heart and blood vessels), respiratory (lungs), muscular (muscles), skeletal (bones), genitourinary (reproductive and urination), digestive (stomach, intestines, etc.), lymphatic (immune), integumentary (skin), and endocrine (glandular) systems. I even asked about the mental, emotional, social, and spiritual well-being of the patient. I was shocked the first time I got a form back and found a check in nearly every box. I was even more surprised when similar forms were handed in on a constant basis. Patients would tell me, "Dr. Senne, everything hurts, I'm depressed, and what doesn't hurt doesn't work."

In those early days of practice, I specialized in joint and muscular problems, and most notably "bad" backs. I would look at all those checked boxes on the symptom survey form and feel sorry for those patients. All I could do was say a silent prayer and hope that in the future, the patients would somehow feel better. I was a back specialist. How in the world was I going to relieve the myriad of symptoms that these people were experiencing? How could *any* doctor help them?

Whenever a new patient entered my clinic, I spoke to him at length. Often, the patient had just been told by another physician that his body was not functioning properly. I would ask, "What did that doctor tell you to do to get well?" Usually, the doctor had told him that he would have to live with the problem, which was a chronic condition, or that he would have to use a medication to control the symptoms indefinitely. Naturally, the patient was often distraught.

As I learned more about the health problems facing my patients, I began to rethink my practice. I wanted to understand why there were so many sick and diseased people in our society. Did good health essentially depend on a roll of the dice? Were a lot of people simply destined to end up in assisted care facilities and nursing homes? Or was something causing so many people to suffer poor health, and could this "something" be avoided?

I reasoned that there must be basic common denominators in people's lives that cause them to become sick, suffer degenerative conditions, and perhaps die prematurely. Eventually, I did identify the common denominators (more about that later), and was able to tell my patients how to address the real reasons for their ill health. Although I wanted to alleviate my patients' immediate discomfort, I wasn't interested in treating just the symptoms. My real goal was to identify and correct the root cause of the problem. Once this was done, many or all of a patient's symptoms would go away. In fact, after treatment, many patients would say that besides being rid of the ache or pain that had brought them to my office at the start, they now also slept far better, had greater energy, or were no longer experiencing the stomachaches that had plagued them for so many years. The natural treatments I used had affected the *whole person*—not just the symptoms.

THE COMMON DENOMINATORS

Above, I mentioned that there are common denominators which cause us to be sick and suffer degenerative conditions. What are these common denominators?

The first common cause of ill health is all the toxins that come into our body. Toxins can have an immediate negative effect upon the body, or can accumulate and cause poor health later on in life. When I say "toxins," I am referring to many different substances and even ideas, including harmful organisms such as viruses, bacteria, and parasites; inorganic minerals and other pollutants that are added to our food, water, air, clothes, cosmetics, household cleaners, cooking containers, supplements, and living and working environments; negative information that enters our mind and soul; and unhealthy relationships that affect our emotional well-being. These toxins set the body up for sickness, disease, and degeneration.

The second common denominator that causes ill health is the failure to use the tools needed to detoxify the body and repair and rebuild health. We need to use fasting and regular elimination to help us detoxify. We need proper nutrition, clean water, exercise, sunlight, good posture, and adequate rest to help us repair and rebuild. In addition, we need uplifting and inspiring information, positive relationships, and a purpose-filled life.

My approach to health is threefold. First, I aim to detoxify the body and eliminate the impurities that are clogging your arteries, capillaries, veins, bones, and tissues, as well as your mind and soul. Then, I provide the building blocks that will allow your body to repair and rebuild itself, making you stronger and healthier. Finally, I help you avoid the toxins that cause health problems.

There is so much information and misinformation on health in our society that it is difficult to determine what is significant and what is simply "noise." My goal is to provide an easy step-by-step approach that you can use to attain good health—perhaps for the first time in your life—and then maintain that well-being for many years to come.

WHAT'S IN THIS BOOK

Chapters 1 through 8 of this book discuss what might be called the "pillars" of good physical health. In these chapters, you will learn about the importance of pure water, clean food, once-a-week fasting, gentle exercise, sunlight, good posture, adequate rest, and bowel health. Each discussion not only explains the issue, but also gives you clear guidelines for making healthy changes in your life so that you can immediately begin to experience better health.

Because good physical health is not possible without mental, emotional, spiritual, and social well-being, Chapters 9 through 12 address these important issues. You will learn how to detoxify, repair, and rebuild your mind; how to build better, more satisfying relationships with friends and family; and lastly, how to create a relationship with God that will nourish your spirit throughout your life.

Chapters 13 through 20 each focus on an area that can have an important impact on your life and health. Topics include storing and preparing your food, beauty and hygiene, clothing, household cleaners and the home environment, household electricity and electromagnetic fields, nutritional supplements, integrative and alternative therapies, and minor injuries and illnesses. In each case, you will learn how to avoid practices that can be harmful to your well-being, and how to make choices that can maximize your health.

Chapter 21, "Putting It All Together," shows you how to pull together all that you have learned to create a practical daily routine. It's easier than you think to incorporate my recommendations into a healthy lifestyle.

Please be aware that if you have a health disorder, this book is not intended to replace evaluation by a healthcare professional. However, I do suggest that when you work with a healthcare provider, you make sure to understand the goals and objectives regarding your treatment. You have a right to know and understand a doctor's plan regarding your health, and you have a right to choose a plan of treatment that makes sense to you.

Within these pages, you will find a commonsense approach that can benefit people of all ages, including infants, children, adolescents, adults, and seniors. My hope is that you will use this book as a comprehensive guide to making healthier choices in your life, both for yourself and for your family. Enjoy!

1. Water

Remember when "Don't drink the water" referred to foreign countries?

We live in a country that has an abundant supply of water. For the most part, everyone has access to water for drinking, bathing, washing clothes and dishes, and even watering lawns. But is all this readily available water good for us? All too many people don't think twice about turning on the faucet and drinking a large glass of tap water, but the unfortunate truth is that tap water can contain toxic inorganic minerals, chemicals, and harmful bacteria. The water may be plentiful, but it's not always fit for consumption.

Water makes up 70 percent of the body, and is actually more important than food for survival. Humans can survive without food for a few weeks, but only for three to five days without water. Water is essential for all the cells of the body to work at peak capacity during cell division. It is vital for both proper digestion and proper elimination. In addition, water is crucial for keeping our internal body temperature within its correct range (97°F to 99°F), and is an important lubricant for our organs, joints, muscles, and tissues. It's no wonder that drinking clean water is one of the best ways to attain and maintain our health.

How do we get clean, pure water? Some people say this is accomplished through a process called distillation; others claim that pure water is obtained through a process known as reverse osmosis; while others say that a simple carbon block filter is all that is needed to produce the clean, pure water that we all want. I know of people who tout the benefits of magnetic water, alkaline water, and oxygenated water. Still others claim that we must add minerals to water to provide the "extra" minerals needed for strong bones and teeth.

It's easy to get confused by all the hype regarding this or that type of water. But considering the importance of clean water to your health, it's vital to cut through the hype and take the steps necessary to get the most healthful water available. This chapter will dispel the hype, explain what healthy water is, and guide you in providing wholesome water for yourself and your family.

MINERALS IN YOUR WATER

Earlier in the chapter, I mentioned that some people recommend the use of mineral-rich water. The truth is that you should be getting your *organic minerals* from the foods you eat along with fresh juices from fruits and vegetables. Organic minerals include calcium, magnesium, potassium, zinc, selenium, manganese, and phosphorus, to name a few. These minerals greatly aid in repairing and rebuilding the body.

The minerals you get from tap water are *inorganic minerals* such as sodium chloride, sodium fluoride, aluminum, and lead. These minerals tend to calcify, causing plaque to develop in the body and creating a host of degenerative conditions. I like to compare drinking tap water to taking a walk behind a smoky bus. Walking is good for you just as drinking water is good for you, but the toxins you take in along the way are far from beneficial.

One of the goals in attaining and maintaining your health is to have an internally clean body, free from all the inorganic mineral deposits and other toxins that are so prevalent in our water supply. To prevent sickness, disease, and degeneration, you have to avoid these toxins. As the number of inorganic minerals and other toxins present in our drinking water increases, so does the number of chronic diseases that attack the body. The human body is an amazingly efficient instrument that can handle its share of abuse over time. But not even the human body can maintain health when it is constantly being subjected to toxic substances.

Water acts as a great carrier by helping to transport nutrients to all the cells and organs of the body. But when the water contains inorganic minerals, they get transported to the organs as well. This stresses the organs and results in a host of problems, including arthritis, osteoporosis, kidney stones, liver disease, problem skin, loss of flexibility in muscles, and heart disease.

CALCIFICATION

The human body is made up of a great transport system that includes arteries, veins, and capillaries. Calcification, which is the hardening of tissue through the impregnation of calcium or calcium salts, occurs in these areas of the body due to the drinking of toxic water. Under ideal conditions, the toxins are picked up by the bloodstream, filtered through the liver and kidneys, and flushed out. If the blood vessels become stiff with calcification and the liver and kidneys become hardened and clogged, they are unable to filter out the toxins, leading to ill health. For that reason, clean water is one of the most effective and inexpensive forms of healthcare.

STAYING YOUNG

All of us, regardless of age, want to look and feel young, and the key to holding onto our youthful health is being internally clean. This means being free from the inorganic minerals that keep our organs from functioning properly. Our Creator blessed most of us with a healthy body at birth. He designed us to go through life with a healthy body, mind, and soul, and with social and emotional well-being. The inorganic minerals present in tap water make us age both internally and externally, causing us to feel and look old well before our time. I want my children and grandchildren to see me as a good model of health. I want to be able to play and to *feel* like playing with my loved ones for the rest of my life.

About Contaminants

Environmental Science Technology printed an article on water contaminants stating: "Any contaminant can cause damage if exposure to it creates high concentrations within a cell, and if accumulated, cellular damage can result in disease or death."[1] That is what I have been sharing with you.

HARMFUL LIQUIDS

So far, this chapter has discussed only water as a beverage, but for too many people, water is not the beverage of choice. Instead, they drink soda pop, coffee, fruit juices, and milk. Many of these beverages contain harmful substances. Soda pop is full of acid and sugar, and coffee is usually made with tap water, which, as you now know, is laden with harmful inorganic minerals. Are store-bought fruit juices better? I recommend that you stay away from these juices because they are full of sugar and preservatives. (I will speak about fresh juices a little later in the book.) I also recommend that you avoid pasteurized milk and pasteurized milk products, as the pasteurization process makes the nutrients in milk less available to the body. None of these popular drinks is a substitute for pure, clean water.

HEALING LIQUIDS

People who drink clean water and fresh additive-free fruit and vegetable juices have better functioning, healthier bodies than those who drink other beverages, including tap water. These people feel more vibrant throughout the day and have more energy, improved circulation, and superior memory capability. I have had patients whose joints ached from years of drinking tap water. When they switched to clean water, their aches and pains slowly disappeared.

Clean drinking water also gives the body a strong defense against viral and bacterial infections. People who drink pure water simply do not get sick as often as those who put less than optimal fluids in their body.

What type of water should you be drinking? The two best kinds are reverse osmosis water and steam-distilled water.

MAKING WATER PURE

Water from chemically treated water systems is often contaminated with harmful chemicals and other substances. The water traveling through the copper piping found in many homes can also be loaded with excessive metals that are picked up from the pipes. What can you do to turn this water into a clean, healthful beverage?

Filtration through reverse osmosis (RO) is one excellent way to get pure drinking water. In a reverse osmosis system, tap water is squeezed through a GAC (granulated activated carbon) filter or through several carbon filters that are generally set up under your kitchen counter. I like to call this type of water "fresh squeezed" since it is literally pushed through the filters. The purpose is to have the filters trap the inorganic minerals, bacteria, and chemicals that are common in today's drinking water, thereby providing clean and pure water. The one caveat with reverse osmosis systems is that the filters vary widely in their ability to trap the inorganic solids and harmful bacteria.

The more filtration the water goes through before you drink it, the cleaner the water becomes. At the minimum, an RO system should consist of a three-stage filter, but a five-stage system is an even better way of ensuring that all the impurities are removed from the water. Because the filters become clogged with impurities over time, and because they are constantly wet and can breed unhealthy bacteria, they need to be changed approximately every six months. But as long as you change the filters regularly, reverse osmosis water is a much better option than unfiltered tap water. For even more protection, you can install an ultraviolet light, which uses light in the UVC range to treat the water after the filtration process, killing any harmful bacteria that remain. The resulting water is much like fresh underground water.

Another good option is a steam-distilling system. In this system, tap water is simply poured into a distiller, and heat is used to vaporize the water. As the steam rises, undesirable substances such as inorganic minerals are left behind in the distiller. The vapor/steam is then sent through a carbon block filter to "capture" any possible inorganic material and bacteria that may remain. The steam condenses and becomes pure water, which drips into a container that doubles as a storage device.

The process of steam distillation is much like the natural process through which rainwater is produced. In Nature, the sun heats up surface water, which evaporates, rises, and condenses in the clouds. When it rains, the water that streams down is—under ideal circumstances—clean and pure. Unfortunately, in our polluted environment of smog and smoke, the rainwater is often contaminated before it hits the ground.

A steam-distilling system ensures that harmful bacteria and other common pollutants are removed from the water. For this reason, steam-distilled water is my preferred choice of drinking water. There is absolutely no truth to the claim that distilled water is "dead" water, or that it leaches vitamins and minerals from the body. These myths are usually spread by people who are marketing their own water-purification systems.

WATER STORAGE

If you opt for a home steam-distilling system, you will then have to store the water it produces. The best choice is a container made of polycarbonate plastic or glass.

Steam-distilled water—*any* water, for that matter—can leach (absorb) toxic chemicals from the plastics commonly used to store it. One such toxic chemical is called bisphenol-A. Used in many plastics, bisphenol-A has been linked to endocrine dysfunction, which results in a host of health problems, including infertility and stunted sexual maturation. The distilled water from a convenience/grocery store is sold in inexpensively made plastic jugs that can easily cause bisphenol-A and similar toxins to leach into your water.

The problem of leaching chemicals is one reason I am not a big proponent of bottled drinking water, but there are other reasons as well. Bottled water can contain contaminants other than plastic chemicals. According to an article cited by the Natural Resources Defense Council, "Some bottled water contains bacterial contaminants." The article then stated, "Chemicals from plastics, or trihalo-methanes—the by-product of the chemical reaction between chlorine and organic matter in water . . . are found in at least some bottles."[2] There is also a big difference between the taste of water stored in a convenience store plastic jug and that of water stored in polycarbonate plastic or glass containers. The taste of properly stored water is far superior.

You may wonder why I recommend polycarbonate plastics as a storage material. The toxic chemical bisphenol-A can be found in polycarbonate plastics

just as it is in most plastics. In more cheaply made plastic containers, the leaching of chemicals is pronounced whether or not the containers are heated. But
due to the nature of polycarbonate, the toxin does not leach out of the container
unless the container is heated. Clearly, this is not too much of a concern with
polycarbonate bottled water. It is, however, an issue when plastics are used to
make baby bottles, which are often heated, causing the chemicals to enter the
baby's formula. A report published by Environment and Human Health, Inc.
stated that there is "Increasing evidence that they [plastics] disrupt normal
growth and development in many different species of animals due to their hormonal activity." The article concluded, "Our youngest will continue to be
exposed, until the federal government adopts and implements a national standard that is protective of children's health."[3] This is why I recommend glass or
polyamide plastic bottles for infants.

Polycarbonate bottles are well worth the minimal investment needed to
safely store the water you drink. If you choose to buy your steam-distilled water,
make sure that the container is made of polycarbonate plastic. If you are using
a home steam distiller, collect the water in the polycarbonate water bottle that
generally comes with the distiller.

WHOLE-HOUSE WATER FILTRATION SYSTEMS

Just as your drinking water should be purified, the water you use for showering, bathing, and washing clothes and dishes should also be filtered. A whole-
house filtration system, also called a point-of-entry filter system, is an excellent
means of removing most of the inorganic minerals and chemicals found in tap
water, making it safe for use. Although this system will not produce water as
clean and pure as the best drinking water, it will make your body, your clothes,
and your dishes look and feel cleaner.

The whole-house system is attached to your incoming water supply line,
usually on the outside of your home or inside your garage. The system is basically just one tank about four feet high and one foot in circumference. The water
is forced through a carbon filter, which needs to be replaced about every five
years. I recommend a GAC (granulated activated carbon) filter, and suggest that
a material called KDF (Kinetic Degradation Fluxion) be installed along with the
carbon. This extra copper-and-zinc filter prevents bacteria from forming inside
the tank. The only drawback to this extra filter is the cost, as it is a bit more
expensive than carbon by itself.

If you do not choose to invest in a whole-house filtration system, the next
best option is to install showerheads that include carbon filters. The filter in each
showerhead is relatively inexpensive and usually needs to be replaced just once

a year. If you take baths rather than showers, you can hang a bathtub filter over your faucet to keep toxic substances out of your bathwater.

If you choose to use a filtered showerhead, look for a device that contains the extra KDF filter so that the water is first filtered through a carbon filter, much like a whole-house filter, and then through the KDF filter. A small shower KDF filter is well worth the few extra dollars it costs, and is far more affordable than a whole-house KDF filter. I personally use both a carbon whole-house water filtration system and KDF filtered showerheads. To minimize costs, rather than having a separate KDF filter for my whole-house system, I have the water dealer mix in some KDF with my carbon.

If you do opt for a point-of-entry whole-house system, make sure the salesperson doesn't talk you into adding a water softener. My salesperson urged me to add a water softener to my filtration unit. Sales must have been slow that month! I not only saved myself a lot of money by not installing a water softener, but I didn't wind up showering or bathing in all the salt that is used to make the water soft. When we shower, bathe, or swim, the body absorbs water through the skin's pores. Moreover, when we breathe during a shower or when we swim in a pool, toxic impurities such as trihalomethanes (a chlorine vapor by-product) enter the body. How harmful are these substances? An article in the *American Journal of Epidemiology* concluded, "Bladder cancer has been associated with exposure to chlorination by-products in drinking water, and experimental evidence suggests that exposure also occurs through inhalation and dermal absorption."[4] We don't need to absorb toxic impurities from our water.

TWO MAJOR WATER TOXINS

Fluoride was first introduced into our drinking water to prevent tooth decay. When isolated from Nature, fluoride is a toxic inorganic mineral that does harden the teeth, but at a cost to the body. You see, fluoride indiscriminately hardens other areas of the body, as well. When fluoride is combined with sodium to produce sodium fluoride, and then added to drinking water, the body experiences a host of health problems. For example, the soft tissues and great transport system (arteries, veins, and capillaries) harden. This is commonly called atherosclerosis, or hardening of the arteries. Poor old cholesterol gets blamed for this, but it is tap water that often causes this problem. Your tissues need to be soft and pliable. When you age, you naturally become less flexible. Your muscles and joints become less supple along with your internal organs, tissues, and transport system. Your skin naturally loses its collagen, causing it to weaken and wrinkle. Fluoride can accelerate the internal hardening of the body, as well as the breakdown of collagen in the skin. The ill effects of fluoride are becoming more apparent. An article published in *The Biological Trace Elements Research Journal* stated that researchers found "a consistent and strong association between the exposure to fluoride and low IQ."[5] I, for one, need all the IQ I can get!

You should eat healthy foods with natural, organic fluoride and drink healthy liquids that will harden your teeth naturally with no possible side effects. If you use organic minerals as Nature intended, and you keep the inorganic minerals out of your body, you will be so much healthier. By adding fluoride to municipal water, scientists attempted to achieve a noble goal but created a health disaster!

Chlorine is another toxic chemical used in our water supply. Chloride is found naturally in Nature and is an important organic mineral used by the body to help regulate metabolism. But when chloride is combined with sodium to produce sodium chloride, toxicity develops and can result in hardening of the arteries along with high blood pressure. When chloride is subjected to electrolysis, chlorine is produced. Chlorine was first introduced as a sanitizer for our water supply. It does a good job of killing many forms of bacteria, which is why it is commonly used in swimming pools. However, chlorine is toxic to the liver and has been known to cause a myriad of health problems.

Journal Report

An article printed in the *American Journal of Public Health* stated that there is "a positive association between consumption of chlorination by-products in drinking water and bladder and rectal cancer in humans."[6] Thanks, but no thanks to that glass of tap water!

One of the major issues with chlorine is that it can kill off the natural "friendly" bacteria that live in the body and automatically fight off harmful bacteria. This destruction of good bacteria greatly suppresses the immune system, leading to numerous health problems down the road. That is why, as mentioned earlier, you need to filter your water through reverse osmosis or steam distillation before you drink it, and use a carbon or KDF filter when you shower or bathe. Once again, scientists had good intentions for the use of chlorine, but water can more safely be sanitized through distillation or the use of ultraviolet light.

SWIMMING POOL AND SPA WATER

If you are a swimmer, I suggest that you swim in a non-chlorinated pool that uses a silver-, ozone-, or titanium-based purification system. These technologies do a nice job of disinfecting pools. Although most public pools and spas still utilize

JENNY—A CASE STUDY

Jenny, a new patient, was a shy individual who was suffering from a case of the blues. She was in her mid-twenties and had recently graduated from college. Although her head and shoulders were slumped forward, she managed to show some enthusiasm when describing her new apartment. Jenny explained that she wasn't always so sad but that she suffered from a lot of aches and pains, which made her depressed. She came to my clinic with a myriad of physical symptoms. The symptom survey form had a lot of checks in those boxes, and another healthcare practitioner had previously diagnosed her as having fibromyalgia, which simply means muscle pain. This reminded me of the doctor who once used a fancy medical term to state that I had a sore foot—as if I didn't already know that! Jenny felt like she was getting the runaround and that nobody really wanted to take the time to help her.

I asked Jenny what kind of water she was drinking. She said that a friend had told her she needed to drink more water, so she had increased the amount of tap water she consumed each day in the hopes of feeling better. Meanwhile, her aches and pains were getting worse, not better, over time. I commended Jenny for drinking water, but explained all that water from her tap was stressing her kidneys and calcifying her arteries. I told Jenny that she needed to start drinking clean, healthy water, which would flush out her body and cleanse her cells.

Jenny mentioned that darkened water rings had formed in her drinking cups. "I thought this was a good way to get my minerals," she said. I explained that those "rings" of inorganic minerals were settling into her body. She said her parents had always used tap water. She saw them every week in a nursing home; sometimes they remembered her and sometimes they didn't. Did the tap water cause their ill health? I'm sure it didn't help. An article published in Environmental Review stated, "The epidemiological evidence indicates that a true association between drinking water aluminum concentrations and dementia (including Alzheimer's disease) cannot be ruled out . . . Aluminum in drinking water is a public health issue."[7]

I recommended that Jenny drink steam-distilled water and that she shower or bathe with a simple shower/bath filter so her body wouldn't absorb all the toxic impurities in the water. She also needed to start a detoxification process to rid herself of the noxious chemicals that had already accumulated in her body.

Following chiropractic treatment to help alleviate her symptoms, Jenny started drinking clean water. She also replaced her old showerhead with a new filtered showerhead. When I saw Jenny three months later, she told me that her muscle aches and joint pains had disappeared. Her head was up and her shoulders were back. I hardly recognized her because she presented herself with so much confidence. Jenny understood the importance of drinking and showering in clean water.

chlorine for disinfection, there is a grass-roots effort to ban chlorine from public pools and spas, and health departments are starting to respond to public concern. Speak with your local pool/spa management and tell them about the hazards posed by chlorine, as well as the money they can save on chemicals by switching to another type of sanitation system. Even if operators used just 50-percent fewer chemicals, swimming pools would pose far less of a health risk, and swimmers would experience no more red eyes, itchy skin, chemical-induced breathing problems, and chemical-induced allergies.

Journal Report

An interesting side note in *Occupational and Environmental Medicine* stated, "It is postulated that increased exposure of children to chlorination products in indoor pools might be an important cause of the rising incidence of childhood asthma and allergic diseases in industrialized countries."[8] May I suggest that this includes outdoor pools as well!

If you have a backyard pool or spa, I suggest checking out the sanitation systems mentioned above, as they will work well to disinfect the water. Swimming in oceans, clean lakes, and ponds is a wonderful alternative to a pool full of chlorine. Ocean swimming is one of the best and healthiest forms of exercise. Watch out for the marine life, though—especially the bigger ones higher up on the food chain!

WATER AS A HEALER

Clean, pure water can benefit you by regulating your bodily functions, including the process of eliminating toxins and body waste. Clean water is the greatest elixir for all the organs, veins, capillaries, arteries, muscles, nerves, bones, and tissues of the body. I recommend drinking six to eight 8-ounce glasses of pure water every day. If you like, squirt a dash of lemon juice into your water. This enhances the water's taste as well as its ability to detoxify the body.

Water is also a very potent healer. I routinely settle into a nice, warm bath in the evening just to relax and unwind. We all know how the warmth of the water makes us feel. If you like to use hot tubs or soak in your own tub, please use clean water and not water that is loaded with chemicals. When you experience sprains and strains, a quick form of water therapy is taking a warm shower for a few minutes followed by a cool shower for a minute or so. This warming and cooling has a tonic effect that is wonderfully refreshing. Alternating warm and cool water also increases circulation in the skin and scalp. (See page 207 in Chapter 20 for more information on treating sprains and strains.)

I am a great advocate of shower therapy. I recommend that when you are in the shower, you simply put some shampoo into the palms of your hands, work up a lather, and proceed to massage your lymphatic glands. Located on the sides of the neck, under the armpits, and down the inside of the legs, the lymphatic glands are among the body's first lines of defense in fighting off infections. These glands contain white blood cells, and it is these cells that are called upon to combat viral and, at times, bacterial infections. The lymphatic glands also help to detoxify the body by circulating body fluids throughout your system. When you massage these glands, you greatly aid lymph circulation and prevent the glands from becoming sluggish or stagnant. The greater a person's illness, the greater the likelihood that the lymphatic system has impaired circulation.

When I shower, I place the fingers of my right hand on the left side of my neck, and gently move my hand downward to my collarbone. I repeat this procedure with my left hand on the right side of my neck. I then take my right hand, cross it over to the left armpit, and move it downwards from the armpit to the waist. I repeat this maneuver with my left hand on the right side of my body. I move my right hand into my left groin, down to the inside of my left thigh, and down to the inside of my left knee. I repeat this procedure with my left hand, except that before I slide my hand to the groin, I move it toward my belly button, stopping about halfway between the waist and the belly button. This movement massages the ileocecal valve, which you'll learn about in Chapter 8. The whole routine takes less than a minute to complete, and is a powerful way to get a sluggish lymph system moving and keep toxins from settling in. As an aside, I also use a loofah sponge and gently rub it over myself to remove any dead skin, as skin cells continually replace themselves. This removal of old skin is another way to help the skin detoxify itself. Finally, I run cool water for a minute or so to wake up my circulatory system.

And So It Was Said . . .

"Water is life's mater and matrix, mother and medium. There is no life without water."
—ALBERT SZENT-GYÖRGYI, 1937
NOBEL PRIZE WINNER FOR PHYSIOLOGY AND MEDICINE

CONCLUSION

You get only one body in your lifetime. Doesn't it make sense to take care of it? One of the reasons people fear getting older is they see many health-challenged seniors and hope that their health doesn't deteriorate to the point where they are in the same situation. Let's not just hope! If you want to get healthy and stay healthy, you must not disregard the rules of Mother Nature. One of her most important rules is to drink clean water. I implore you not to wait until you are suffering ill health to start drinking and using pure water. If you are already experiencing a health crisis, I urge you to take the first step towards wellness by using the best water available.

Your birthright is physical, mental, emotional, social, and spiritual health! Clean water and a clean, well-functioning body go hand in hand. The majority of people simply cannot live a long and healthy life if they don't utilize pure, clean water for drinking and bathing, for it is this water that flushes the toxins out of the body. The truth is that pure water is one of your greatest sources of wealth. There, that was easy! You have begun the first step on the road to great health.

Remember, Health is Wealth!

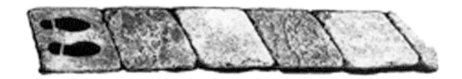

2. Food

Why are there so many malnourished people in the richest country?

We live in a wonderful country with so many opportunities for each and every one of us. We are also blessed by an abundance of food, but is it the kind of food that promotes good health? Why are sickness, disease, and degeneration continuing to climb in the richest nation on earth? Why are obesity and malnourishment at an all-time high? The answer lies in the food we eat.

We should be eating unadulterated, clean foods that are not contaminated by pollutants, not "created" by man, and not modified by man to preserve shelf life. Processed foods are designed to last longer in the supermarket in the hopes that someone will eventually purchase them. They certainly last a long time, but they are not what we should take into our bodies. Instead, we must eat our food in its most natural, clean form so that we get all the nourishment we need, including vitamins, minerals, amino acids, enzymes, and the other substances required by the body for proper metabolism. It's a common myth that we can eat whatever we want as long we take a vitamin and mineral supplement during the day, just in case some nutrient is missing from our food. It's like a vitamin insurance policy in a pill. The use of nutritional supplements along with other dietary potions and formulas are at a record high in this country. These products, however, cannot replace natural, clean food.

CERTIFIED ORGANIC FOODS

What is clean food? Clean food is food that is *certified organic*. Organic plants are raised in clean soil without the use of chemical pesticides, insecticides, and herbicides. Organic meat comes from animals raised on organic land and given organic feed. This is the healthiest food that you can eat. It is high in nutrients because it grows in nutrient-rich soil. A farmer can tell you that if earthworms are present in the soil, the food is good to eat. Earthworms tend not to live in polluted soil. If an earthworm won't live in a certain soil, why would I want to eat foods grown in that soil?

Some people think of organic food as being "weird" or very different from "normal" food. Actually, it is the same food that is found in your local grocery store, except that it is higher in nutrients and free of harmful chemicals. No toxic synthetic fertilizers were used in its cultivation. Instead, the fertilizers used were green manure and compost. The food itself was not sprayed with toxic, synthetic chemicals (organophosphates, carbamates, and bipyridyls) to lengthen its shelf life, nor was it subjected to irradiation (ionizing radiation) to kill off any "bugs." Organic food is also not a genetically modified organism (GMO). Non-organic soybeans and corn are often genetically modified to make them more resistant to the pests that eat crops. Gee, if a bug won't eat the food, maybe that food isn't fit for human consumption, either!

When growing organic produce, farmers use crop rotation and nutrient-rich soil to produce strong, healthy plants that resist destruction by pests and diseases. Organic food not only is high in nutrients and toxin-free, but provides an added benefit as well. The living microorganisms in the soil actually migrate into the food. While this may sound disgusting, soil organisms are beneficial for us to ingest. They actually help preserve our health by building up natural "friendly" bacteria in the body, which in turn fights off illnesses such as bacterial infections.

Defining Organic

The word "organic" is applied not only to naturally grown crops, but also to animals that are fed organic grains and grasses—feed that does not contain synthetic hormones such as testosterone and progesterone, or antibiotics such as penicillin and tetracycline. Unadulterated, non-pasteurized, non-homogenized milk, cheese, and eggs are also considered "organic."

Organic foods may cost a little more due to the stricter regulations governing the certification process, as well as the extra labor needed to stave off pests and disease without chemicals. However, the nutritional benefits far outweigh the slight increase in cost. According to a recent article published by The Organic Center, "Forging a new relationship with food is the critical first step that every dietitian, doctor, educator, and concerned friend is searching for as they interact with a person headed toward, or already contending with, overweight and diabetes." The article continues, "It [organic food and farming] exposes people to fewer of the endocrine disrupting chemicals that can set off the disease process and promote and trigger epigenetic changes. It also delivers higher daily intake of health-promoting phyto (plant) chemicals that reinforce the body's defense and repair mechanism."[1] So try to eat clean food!

Human beings are meant to eat food that is "complete," meaning that it includes a full complement of vitamins, minerals, enzymes, and other nutrients, many of which science has yet to identify and formulate into a pill. Whole foods contain far more nutrition than a vitamin or mineral pill will ever come close to offering. The purpose of eating whole, nutrient-rich foods is to repair and rebuild the body. Refined foods—white flour and sugar, for instance—just don't have the nutritional capacity to repair and rebuild. In fact, these foods are devoid of most or all of their original nutrients. In Chapter 1, I stated that clean, pure water is the great toxin flusher for the body. Clean food that has all its nutrients intact not only detoxifies the body, but is also the great body repairer and rebuilder. I sincerely wonder whether taking vitamin and mineral supplements isn't actually creating more harm rather than good for the body. Even if some supplements don't harm us, we get little benefit from them. I do not want to bank my health on the latest vitamin or mineral pill on the market. Remember, I am speaking about a lifestyle—not about taking another pill.

Recently, I shopped at a local health food store for organic ingredients to make bread. I noticed how many people were filling their shopping carts with bottles of expensive pills, while beside the pills was an assortment of non-organic foods such as white processed flour and sugar—products that I wouldn't feed to a billy goat! I couldn't help but think that a bottle of pills cannot make up for all of that nutrient-poor food.

FRESH MARKETS AND SUPERMARKETS

If you don't have access to organic foods or have a garden of your own, it is likely that there is a farmers' market of some kind nearby. These markets are becoming more common in most communities. While the foods available at these markets are not certified as chemical-free, at least they are not generally sprayed with chemicals. Therefore, the food itself is healthier. If you do buy fruits and vegetables from your local supermarket, and it is not certified organic, please make sure to wash the produce with a hydrogen peroxide-water solution, or to at least scrub it with a hard-bristle brush and rinse off the chemicals as best you can. Hydrogen peroxide is an excellent cleaner of fruits and vegetables and is very healthy for the human body. In fact, many alternative healthcare clinics utilize a diluted form of hydrogen peroxide as oxygen therapy for their patients. An article published in the *American Journal of Epidemiology* stated, "Lower cognitive performance was observed in subjects who had been occupationally exposed to pesticides."[2] I guess I won't be eating those shiny, waxed supermarket apples!

If a food is advertised as being all-natural, it is not supposed to contain any additives—according to the advertiser, that is. The food, however, has not been checked by a certifying agency. When a food is certified organic, on the other hand, both the soil it was grown in and the food itself has been inspected.

One of the advantages of certain fruits and vegetables is that they have a natural covering, providing some protection from the chemicals used in their cultivation. For example, produce such as melons, bananas, oranges, pineapple, and corn has tough skins or husks that are removed before the food is eaten. By eliminating the covering, you eliminate much of the chemical spray used in the growing process. Produce such as grapes, strawberries, pears, apples, berries, carrots, and beets has no protective covering besides a very thin peel. And unfortunately, when you remove the peel, you remove the most nutrient-rich portion of the food.

All produce that has no protective covering should be organic since it is difficult, if not impossible, to remove the chemicals that have been sprayed onto and absorbed into the food. If your produce is non-organic, it should be washed in clean water and—if it has a hard consistency, like carrots—scrubbed with a brush. I still prefer organic vegetables and fruit, not only because of the nutritionally rich soil in which it is grown, but also because no chemicals have been absorbed by the food.

There was a time not long ago when I lived in an area of the country where I was limited in my selection of organic foods, so I know it's not always easy to find. Do what you can. If you can't find an organic or farmers' market, and you do not have your own garden, you have no choice but to shop at your local grocery store and scrub your produce clean. At the end of this book, I have included a Resources section listing companies that offer organic foods.

A STANDARD MEAL PLAN

Most people should eat the standard three meals a day. What is a standard three-meal-a-day plan? Everyone likes to eat in their own manner. However, you should incorporate some type of fruit or vegetable, either in solid or juiced form, into each meal, preferably at the beginning of the meal. This will greatly benefit your health.

Fruits and vegetables do an excellent job of preparing the digestive and elimination system for the other foods that follow during your meal. They are also loaded with a host of nutrients.

I suggest eating meat no more than three times per week, and my reasoning is twofold. First, because of meat's inherent fat content—yes, even lean meats have fat—the body's transport system (blood vessels) tends to be clogged by a diet rich in meat. Second, the digestive and elimination systems have to work harder to process meat than they do to process fruits, vegetables, grains, and even dairy products. It's simply more difficult to break meats down. Since it is more work for the stomach to break down meat, meat often fails to be completely digested, and the undigested meat is passed into the colon and stored for a longer period of time than occurs with fruit and vegetables. This means that less nutrition is absorbed by the body. It really boils down to what we can absorb. I'll talk about digestion and elimination in much more detail later on in the book.

THE DIET

The human diet should be focused on fresh fruits and vegetables. Fruits are loaded with vitamins, which act as a cleanser/detoxifier for the body, and vegetables are full of minerals, which act as a body repairer and rebuilder. The three main reasons for illness and degeneration are the toxic buildup in the body; the inability of the body to flush, repair, and rebuild itself; and the failure to avoid the toxins that caused the disorders in the first place. Good nutrition and organic foods, when available, are excellent ways of helping the body detoxify, repair, and rebuild.

Following fruits and vegetables and their respective juices, a healthful diet is formed by organic whole grains (wheat, barley, millet, flax, and rice); nuts; seeds (raw and unsalted) and their butters (almond and sesame butter); beans and legumes; meat (beef, venison, fowl, and fish); dairy products (unprocessed milk, kefir, and cheese); eggs; and natural oils (olive, flax, and coconut). Many people opt to soak their seeds and nuts overnight in clean water, dry them, soak them again, and dry them again before eating them a couple of days later. The purpose is to simply soften up the seeds and nuts to aid in digestion. Soaking also supports the germination process (sprouting) of the seed and nut. You can even drink the water that the seeds and nuts were soaked in. Some folks enjoy eating fermented vegetables such as sauerkraut. (I do not like the taste of sauerkraut, but more power to you if you do.) Sauerkraut is a very healthy food and acts much like a probiotic in building up the body's "friendly" bacteria.

JUICING

Juicing is an excellent way to get our fruits and veggies for the day. I love to eat fruit but I have never really enjoyed eating vegetables—not even salads. By simply tossing several different types of organic fruits (with the seeds) or vegetables (with the leaves and stems) into my juicer, I can consume a large glass of fresh body-cleansing fruit juice or body-repairing vegetable juice with no preservatives. I generally have a fresh glass of fruit juice in the morning. Later in the day, I place an assortment of vegetables in my juicer, add an apple to sweeten it a bit, and drink a glass of vegetable juice. Vegetables are the great body repairers and rebuilders, and fruits are the great body cleansers. In fact, the only liquids I generally drink are clean, pure steam-distilled water and fresh fruit and vegetable juices. If for some reason I miss juicing for a day, I try to drink six to eight 8-ounce glasses of clean water. I usually drink about four 8-ounce glasses of water on the days I juice.

Unless I am traveling, I aim to drink a couple of glasses of juice per day. Juicing is extremely healthy, and juicers are rather inexpensive and readily available in any store that offers kitchen products. Fresh non-pasteurized juice is loaded with vitamins, minerals, enzymes, and all the cofactors that make for a complete nutritional drink. Juicing can be started with your children as early as two years of age. By that time, kids have usually been introduced to a wide variety of foods, and their digestive, absorption, and elimination systems are better able to handle the nutrient rush provided by juices.

Juicing is a very easy and efficient way to instantly put nutrients into the bloodstream. The bloodstream carries the nutrients to all the cells to detoxify, repair, and rebuild the body. The body does not have to break down the fruits and vegetables since the juicer has already taken care of that.

The more sick, diseased, and degenerated my patients were, the more I would stress the importance of a juicing program. Many diabetic patients worried that their bodies could not handle juicing because the naturally occurring sugars in the juice would spike their blood sugar levels. I suggested that those patients dilute the juice with water, or use a blender in place of a juicer so that the fiber of the produce was retained. The fiber then slowed the body's absorption of the juice.

Whether juicing or blending, I have found that including the seeds in the fruits and vegetables makes the drink even more beneficial. The seeds are full of the right balance of nutrients that the body needs to help regulate its hormones. Fruits and vegetables with seeds intact are called "live" foods. These foods are capable of reproducing. Have you ever planted a watermelon seed and watched it grow into a watermelon? Such foods can reproduce because they are loaded with all the healthful cofactors that science has yet to discover and cannot duplicate in pill form. It should be noted, however, that the pits of most fruits simply can't be broken down by a juicer or blender, and therefore must be discarded.

Many people seek out fruits and vegetables that are seedless so that they don't have to "deal" with seeds. However, this produce is often a crossbred, altered food whose nutritional value pales compared with that of seed-bearing fruits and vegetables.

The Importance of Seed-Bearing Fruits

Many religious books talk about the importance of eating seed-bearing fruits and vegetables. For example, Genesis 1:29 states, "Then God said, 'I give you every seed-bearing plant on the face of the whole earth and every tree that has fruit with seed in it.'"
—NEW INTERNATIONAL VERSION HOLY BIBLE

I also enjoy adding sprouted grains to my diet. The sprouts refer to the "seed" of the grain. The green part of fruits and vegetables, such as the leaves and stems, contain chlorophyll, which is also very healthful. Chlorophyll binds with the hemoglobin in our red blood cells to increase the oxygen supply in the body. I have personally found watermelon juice with the seeds ground up to be a wonderful blended juice drink. I often make this beverage when not using my juicer. Yup, seeds and all! It's very easy to do. You simply cut up your favorite fruit, or a variety of fruits, and put it in a blender. The result is a healthful fruit smoothie.

All the cells of the body except for the nerve cells reproduce every day, week, month, and year. This is why it's so important to avoid as many toxins as possible, to drink clean water and juices, and to feed your body whole nutritious foods with the seeds, stems, and leaves still intact whenever possible. This will help ensure that the cells being produced are healthful and function properly.

A general rule is to avoid juicing fruits and vegetables together in the same drink, with the exception of sweetening up your vegetable juice with an apple. If you want to drink both fruit juice and vegetable juice within a short period of time, I advise waiting about fifteen minutes between the drinks. If you consume a lot of different fruit and vegetable juices in the same beverage, you may get a bit of an upset stomach.

MEATS

I would like to briefly discuss the topic of meat. When purchasing meat, it is important to seek out organically fed, antibiotic-free, hormone-free products. I do enjoy eating meat, but due to its inherent fat content, I limit my intake to no more than two servings of meat per week. Beef and venison are good, healthy meats. The one type of meat that one should never eat is pork and its by-products.

Fish also falls into the "meat" category and is much more easily digested than other types of meat. I recommend wild fish, with salmon, cod, and halibut being at the top of my meat-eating list because they tend to have the lowest mercury levels. (Shark, tuna, and swordfish have the highest levels of mercury.) I recommend staying away from farm-raised fish due to their non-organic feed, and I advise you to avoid shellfish such as lobster, clams, and shrimp. These animals are known as bottom feeders because they are the scavengers of the sea, and eat the excrement of the other fish. Yuck! Pigs are much the same as they, too, are scavengers.

When chicken, turkey, and duck are organically fed and antibiotic-free, they also are healthful to eat. Thank goodness it is no longer legal to use hormones in the raising of fowl. If you compare fowl that eats seeds and other wild plant life to birds of prey that eat flesh, you'll find the seed eaters to be much healthier. This brings up a general point about eating meat. Animals that eat the flesh of other animals are not nearly as good for us as animals that eat plants. A cow can get strong and healthy on grass. When we eat that cow, though, we are getting our nutrition *secondhand*. If we eat an animal of prey that has consumed the flesh of another animal, we are getting our nutrition *thirdhand*, because the plant nutrients were eaten by the first animal, which was then eaten by the second animal, which only then was eaten by us. It's far healthier to get our food in the first stage of the nutritional cycle, from fruits, vegetables, and grains. This nutrition is more complete.

This reminds me of a picnic table analogy. Imagine sitting at the end of a picnic table that has lots of other people sitting around it, too. You tell a story to the person beside you, who repeats the story to the person next to him, who then passes it on, etc. By the time the story gets to the other end of the table, it is something very different from what it started out to be.

The animals and people who live the longest generally get their nutrition firsthand from the primary source—the land. That's where you should be getting most of your food.

Many people mistakenly feel that in order to get protein in their diets, they need to eat meat. Actually vegetables, beans, legumes, and whole food supplementation can satisfy all your protein requirements. When you cook your meat, you will greatly diminish the amino acids (protein building blocks) in the food. Therefore, the nutritional value of the meat will be compromised.

Finally, I suggest avoiding processed meats such as luncheon meats and hot dogs, as they contain toxins such as nitrates; smoked meats, which contain nitrosamines; and cured meats, which contain a large quantity of salt as a preservative.

EGGS

You should eat eggs from organically fed, antibiotic-free, free-range fowl. Eggs that are certified organic meet all these requirements. Don't worry about the cholesterol in the egg. In their natural state, the egg white and its yolk are loaded with valuable nutrients and are very good for you. For example, an egg yolk is loaded with essential fatty acids, notably a fatty acid called DHA (docosahexaenoic acid), and cholesterol, both of which are beneficial for the brain. Cholesterol gets a bad rap, but it is vitally important in keeping both the brain and the blood healthy. This is why when you consume products that Nature intended you to eat, you do not need to be concerned about cholesterol, since everyone's cholesterol levels will vary. It is when you consume man-made products that contain hydrogenated and "trans" fats that you need to be worried, because they can cause you to have elevated "bad" cholesterol levels, or increased low-density lipoprotein (LDL). By eating foods such as eggs in their natural state, you are getting the "good" cholesterol, high-density lipoprotein (HDL).

COW'S MILK

It is important to buy milk in its raw, pure, non-pasteurized, and non-homogenized form, just like the milk that our grandparents and many of our parents drank. Raw milk is different from organic milk because organic milk is often pasteurized and homogenized. The pasteurization process does prolong the shelf life of milk and kill off any bacteria that may be present. However, the heating process also destroys much of the nutrition in the milk.

Homogenization is the mechanical process of breaking up the fat (cream) part of the milk and dissolving it into the rest of the milk. The problem with homogenization is that the healthy fat of the milk is beneficial to the body. The fat contains the milk enzyme XO (xanthine oxidase), and when this enzyme is broken down through homogenization, the fat cannot be properly absorbed by the body. The fat then accumulates in your transport system and causes a host of problems such as clogging of the arteries. You should drink whole milk, not skim, 1-percent, or any other manipulated form of milk, as processing diminishes the milk's ability to be used by the body. If you don't have access to raw milk, organic cow's milk is healthier than grocery store milk because it is free from chemicals such as recombinant bovine growth hormone (rBGH).

GOAT'S MILK

Many people are allergic to cow's milk and its by-products, such as cheese and yogurt. Goat's milk and its by-products are far less likely to cause problems. Why? You may know that breast milk is Nature's most complete food for infants. Well, goat's milk is close to human breast milk in both consistency and nutritional composition.

My daughter consumed raw goat's milk after she was weaned off the breast and suffered no ill effects from drinking it, at least not that I am aware of! No, she doesn't howl at the moon at night. When it became difficult to obtain raw goat's milk, I simply switched my daughter to organic apple cider. She wanted milk for her cereal, but when I put apple cider on her cereal, she loved it!

Generally, if you have a good supply of "friendly" bacteria in your body, that bacteria, along with the "friendly" bacteria in the raw milk, will neutralize any "bad" bacteria that may be lingering in the milk, and you will reap the nutritional benefits. For centuries, raw milk was the only milk available. If you think about it, refrigeration and pasteurization have been around for only a few decades.

I suggest giving an infant goat's milk if the infant is not going to be receiving breast milk. It is hard to find raw goat's milk unless you know of a farmer who has goats, but there are companies that supply this type of milk. There are also companies that supply pasteurized goat's milk for people who prefer their milk to be pasteurized. (See page 234 of the Resources section.) When feeding an infant, I suggest diluting the goat's milk with purified water. If the infant can't digest goat's milk, which is rare, try a lactose-free formula.

If your infant is put on milk other than breast milk, and it has been pasteurized, you may want to supplement the milk with one-eighth teaspoon of infant probiotics a day. If the milk has been homogenized, supplement with one-eighth teaspoon of coconut, flaxseed, or olive oil, alternating the oils so that the child receives some of each oil every week. If the milk has been both pasteurized and homogenized, give the child both probiotics and oil. The probiotics will help build up the infant's immune system, and the oils will help with brain and nervous system development. I suggest supplementing one feeding per day.

If your infant is put on formula, you may want to supplement the formula with one-eighth teaspoon of infant probiotics and one-eighth teaspoon of coconut, flaxseed, or olive oil, alternating the oils. While I'm addressing the subject of infant formulas, I'd like to add a caveat. If you do choose to use a formula, try to avoid soy-based products since many contain the additive monosodium glutamate (MSG), which can cause respiratory distress in some infants.

MILK SUBSTITUTES

If you cannot or do not want to drink goat's milk, consider trying rice or almond milk. These milks are delicious and are a great vegetarian alternative. You may have noticed that I haven't mentioned soymilk. Although popular, soymilk and other soy products can cause estrogen-related characteristics in people. It can alter a woman's delicate estrogen balance, causing more hormonal problems, and can have estrogen-like effects on men as well. Estrogen is a hormone that I really don't need any more of in my body, thank you! For this reason, in my practice, I never recommended soymilk to either women or men. I realize that soy products have helped some women manage hormonal issues—hot flashes in particular. It has been my experience, though, that soy products taken for an extended period of time can further upset the hormonal balance of the body.

According to an article offered on Scribd, "This [soy] is particularly detrimental to the health of males as it lowers their level of testosterone, resulting in feminizing effects on masculine features, as well as lower sperm count and decreased sex drive." The article continued, "Despite being hailed as a female-friendly miracle food, due to its ability to mimic the effects of estrogen, soy has also been linked to depression and menstrual irregularities in women."[3] I'm depressed reading about this and I am not even a woman.

THE BENEFITS OF BREAST-FEEDING

As you may have already gathered from the discussion on page 28, I heartily recommend that all infants start out drinking breast milk. I know many mothers who say they don't have the time to breast-feed their children, but the nutrients in breast milk are the most complete nutrition you can give your baby as he begins life. The first few months are so important for the health of the baby. The baby not only gets highly nutritious food from the milk that Mother Nature has intended and provided, but also receives a range of antibodies—proteins in the blood used by the immune system to neutralize bacteria and viruses. These antibodies, as well as other nutritional components offered in breast milk, keep the baby from getting so many of the common sicknesses from which today's infants suffer.

The longer you can breast-feed your baby, the better. Breast-fed babies tend to have higher learning abilities than formula-fed babies because of the essential fatty acids and other cofactors (which are hard to reproduce) supplied in the mother's breast milk. These nutrients are necessary for brain development because the brain is made up of about 60 percent fat.

Journal Report

An article published in *The Journal of the American Medical Association* suggested, "Breastfeeding may have long-term positive effects on cognitive and intellectual development."[4]

I usually recommend that women breast-feed for at least three months. If you can, continue for six months, and even up to a year or more. I have seen mothers nurse their children up to four years of age, which may be going a bit overboard. However, it is certainly not uncommon to have a goal of up to one year of breast-feeding. My wife has never particularly enjoyed breast-feeding, although she hears other mothers say how much they enjoy it. Nevertheless, she does it because she knows the nutritional benefits it has given our daughter and currently gives our son. She feels that one year of inconvenience is well worth the reward of giving her children the best nutritional start in life. It's much like a savings bond of health.

My wife breast-fed our daughter for the first sixteen months of her young life. (She said she was stopping after one year. The year came and went, I didn't say anything, and she kept going.) Our young son is currently being breast-fed. Breast-feeding has not only provided superior nutrition for our children, but also created an incredible bonding experience between mother and baby. Can you tell that I am a big proponent of breast-feeding?

If you wish to breast-feed your child but are having difficulty producing milk, I suggest consuming red raspberry leaf herbal tea. One cup per day— along with the healthy diet discussed throughout this book—is generally all that is needed to aid the body in producing breast milk.

Breast-Feeding Is Healthy for Baby and Mom

Did you know that breast-feeding can result in the mother's breasts staying healthier throughout her lifetime? The highly nutritious milk, full of life-promoting hormones for the baby, flows through the mother's breasts, improving her health as well. As for the infant, breast-feeding is a great way to help develop little facial and head bones since the suckling action is more work for a baby than obtaining milk from a bottle.

BREAST-PUMPING

If you are concerned about a lack of breast milk production when your child is sleeping through the night, I suggest that you obtain a breast pump and pump your milk on a three-hour schedule throughout the night. This continued routine of breast pumping greatly aids any woman who tends to "dry up" earlier than she had hoped. I realize it is an inconvenience to wake up throughout the night and pump, but—provided you get adequate nutrition and rest between pumpings—this will keep the breast milk flowing and even make it possible to bank (freeze) the extra milk pumped during the night.

Breast-pumping is also helpful if you work outside the home. To save time, use a double breast pump. Breast milk can easily be stored in a refrigerator for up to three days and can be frozen for up to three months for later use.

INFANT FEEDINGS

When you are breast-feeding your infant, your infant will generally be satisfied with getting all the milk he needs through the breast. When bottle-feeding your child, you may not know how many ounces to give your infant. Newborn infants generally drink between one to three ounces of milk at a feeding. Between one to two months of age, an infant should be drinking between three to four ounces at one feeding.

Between two to six months of age, an infant should be drinking four to six ounces at a feeding, and between six to twelve months, he should be drinking six to eight ounces at a feeding.

A newborn should have four to six feedings within a twenty-four-hour time period. When the baby is about sixteen weeks of age, the fifth and sixth feedings are usually dropped as he begins to sleep through the night. By this time, the infant should be eating every three and a half to four hours. This feeding schedule should continue even after solid foods have been introduced, usually at about twelve months of age. As the child develops physically and consumes more at each feeding, feedings become farther apart.

When a child wakes up at night, in most cases, either he is wet and needs a diaper change, or he is hungry. Once the diaper has been changed, if he is still fussy, continue with the night feeding until the fussiness is no longer due to hunger. Infants' needs may vary, but this is a good general guideline. Our daughter was breast-fed for several months even after we introduced her to solid foods. She would eat and then get off the breast when she was finished. Our son, on the other hand, would take his sweet time on the breast and would very often fall asleep while eating. The feeding time would take quite a while and he would still be fussy when he finished eating. This didn't make either mother or son too happy. When my wife started to pump her milk and feed it to him via a bottle, he was much happier and the feedings were of shorter duration. Mother and son were satisfied. Don't forget to burp your baby after each feeding. This may sound like a no-brainer, but burping my daughter was something I would occasionally forget to do. She would look at me as if to say, "Dad, aren't you forgetting something?"

Healthy Tips for Storing and Feeding Breast Milk and Formula

If you opt to feed your child formula, or if you pump your own milk and later feed it by bottle, I suggest that you use glass or polyamide bottles. Many plastic bottles, including those made with polycarbonate plastic, can leach plastic into the formula or breast milk when heated. This won't happen with polyamide plastic. Look for silicone nipples and pacifiers versus latex or rubber, as latex and rubber can cause allergic reactions in some infants. When freezing breast milk, use biodegradable food grade plastic bags made of polyethylene or polypropylene. When your infant gets a little older and is ready for training cups, look for cups made of polycarbonate or polyamide plastic.

INTRODUCING YOUR BABY TO HIS FIRST SOLID FOODS

Try to wait at least six months before you give your baby solid foods. Generally, your baby will do just fine on breast milk alone for the first six months of his life. If your infant is receiving formula, please supplement it with oil and probiotics as explained earlier in this chapter, on page 28.

Solid food that is introduced very early in an infant's life can set a little one up for health problems down the road, with food allergies being the most common. This means that as the infant gets older, he will have more difficulty processing his food and will have to avoid certain foods entirely. The infant's digestive tract simply isn't equipped to break down, absorb, and eliminate solid food early in life. The digestive system has to mature, just like the rest of the child. Nature intended babies to have breast milk throughout infancy. Many children are breast-fed exclusively for up to a year before starting solid foods. If you allow their digestive tract time to develop properly, they will enjoy food and experience many fewer food allergy-associated problems over time.

You will know when your breast milk alone will no longer satisfy the child. I mentioned that my daughter started solid foods at ten months of age. My son, who is now ten months old, is still completely satisfied with breast milk alone. When breast milk begins to be insufficient for a child, he will want to continue to suckle past his normal feeding time even when the breast is empty. At that point—when the baby does not seem satisfied after being breast-fed—you should start introducing solid food. However, continue supplementing the infant's diet with breast milk. As I already mentioned, the longer you can breast-feed, the better. I have seen women wearing t-shirts that say "Breast Is Best." I hope they are referring to the milk!

When you first introduce solids, it is best to stick with one type of solid food throughout the day. Grains are the perfect first food for an infant. Whole grain brown rice or millet is easy for an infant to digest, and can be given multiple times throughout the day along with milk or formula. I suggest feeding your infant rice cereal for a week before adding another grain, such as millet. Wait yet another week before adding oatmeal to his diet, and then another week before providing a mixed-grain cereal.

Once your child is used to several grains, you can start adding veggies to his diet. I suggest beginning with steamed yams that have been softened to the proper consistency. At the end of the week, introduce yet another vegetable, such as steamed and softened green beans. Each week, add a new vegetable while continuing to give your child the vegetables and grains that are already part of his diet.

After a month or two of vegetables, introduce blended, softened fruits to your child's diet. I suggest starting with bananas and providing it for one week. Follow this with pears, again, for a week, as you continue to offer grains and vegetables. Every week, add a new fruit.

After a month or two of fruits, mix one-fourth teaspoon of seed or nut butter in with your child's grains a few times a week. You can even add a little oil to the grains around the time you add the butters, alternating about one-fourth teaspoon of butters one day with one-fourth teaspoon of oil the next day. Then introduce cooked beans and legumes, again allowing your child to get used to one food for a week before introducing another.

Don't introduce your child to sweets at an early age. If he begins eating sweets too soon, you will have a much greater problem getting him to eat vegetables and fruits because his taste buds will crave sweets. Wouldn't you rather

Is It Milk Allergy or Milk Intolerance

A lot of people use the terms "milk allergy" and "milk intolerance" synonymously, but they are really two different disorders. When a milk allergy is present, the individual's immune system reacts against the proteins in milk, causing symptoms ranging from breathing difficulties to diarrhea and vomiting. A milk intolerance or lactose intolerance, on the other hand, does not involve the immune system, but occurs when the body is unable to digest the milk. This results in stomach pain, diarrhea, gas, and other symptoms of poor digestion.

eat a cookie than a carrot? If your young child doesn't taste cookies for a few years, he will think that vegetables are great!

INTRODUCING DAIRY AND MEAT TO BABIES

As discussed on page 28, goat's milk is similar to human breast milk in composition. For that reason, it can be introduced into the child's diet at any time. However, cow's milk and cow's milk products—cheese and yogurt, for instance—should not be introduced until the child is sixteen to eighteen months of age. Cow's milk is not like human breast milk, and many children develop an allergy to it if it is introduced too early. This may cause the child to experience further associated health problems, such as asthma, ear infections, and allergies to other foods.

When a child experiences a lot of illness, one of the first things I advise the parents to do is to take him off cow's milk. When cow's milk is eliminated from the diet, sickness—most notably, ear infections and allergies—often disappears. Kids even start to breathe easier.

I suggest that parents avoid introducing meat for up to the first two years of a child's life. Before that time, the digestive tract simply isn't mature enough to break down and absorb meat.

MICHAEL—A CASE STUDY

Michael was brought to my clinic by his parents. He was fourteen years old and desperately wanted to run on his school track team. The only problem was that he couldn't run. There was nothing wrong with his legs—it was his lungs. He had developed asthmatic symptoms, and would start to wheeze after running even a short distance.

When Michael ran around during gym class in the morning, his asthma was not bad. In the afternoon, though, Michael would drink chocolate milk after school and then be unable to run. Michael said he drank the milk just before running because he did not want to get dehydrated and he didn't care too much for plain water.

I told Michael and his parents that his milk-drinking days would have to come to a halt if he wanted to rid himself of his breathing problems. Michael was wheezing because he had a milk allergy, which causes the immune system to react against one or more of the proteins found in milk. "But I can't live without my chocolate milk," Michael stated. "How bad do you want to be on the track team?" I asked. Michael gave up his milk, made the track team, and did quite well.

LIQUIDS WITH MEALS

I do not drink any liquids—not even water or juice—with my meals. Liquids dilute the powerful digestive acids and enzymes we have in our stomach. When we dilute these acids and enzymes, our food is less likely to get broken down, and we are able to extract and absorb less nutrition from it. Furthermore, when liquids are consumed with meals, food is much less likely to be completely eliminated from the body, leading to toxic accumulation. If I have something to drink, I usually wait ten to fifteen minutes before having a meal. Once I've completed a meal, I wait ten to fifteen minutes before drinking my beverage.

I have heard patients say that they need to drink a liquid with their meals in order to "get their food down," or that they get thirsty when they eat, and therefore drink liquid with their food. The solution is simple—they should simply chew their food for a longer period of time. Chewing helps get the digestive juices flowing in the mouth to aid in the breakdown of the food. When people get thirsty while eating, it is often because the food is too salty. Stay away from that salt shaker! (More on salt shortly.)

This is a good time to address the subject of alcohol. My patients often asked, "What if I just have a little red wine with my meals?" Personally, I don't drink alcohol, but if consumed in moderation, I see no harm in it. By "moderation," I mean only a couple of ounces per day. If you do choose to drink alcohol, I suggest that you look for an organic wine, as it will be "cleaner" and contain no pesticides or other toxic chemicals. Wait at least fifteen minutes after finishing your meal before you relax with your wine. This will allow your digestive enzymes to do their work before you dilute them with liquid. Finally, if you are among the many people who cannot handle alcohol, I urge you to avoid it entirely.

Is Non-Alcoholic Beer a Soft Drink?

Although the amount of alcohol in non-alcoholic beer is minimal, there is some alcohol present. Therefore, if you are trying to avoid alcohol, you should definitely skip this beverage.

PH, ACIDITY, AND ALKALINITY

Due to the addition of preservatives and sugar, and to pasteurization, grocery store juices are not a good source of nutrition. Definitely stay away from any liquid found in a can. Soda pop, for instance, is loaded with refined sugar, phosphoric acid, and high fructose corn syrup—all substances that the body doesn't need. Even if you can get soda pop from a bottle, the acid and sugars cause inorganic deposits to form in the joints of the body, leading to pain and stiffness.

The phosphoric acid in soda pop can create ill health in another way, as well. The acid in foods can alter the pH (potential hydrogen) of the blood. Blood has a pH of about 7, and when the pH goes higher than 7, the blood is more alkaline, which generally leads to good health. When blood pH dips below 7, however, the blood becomes more acidic and ill health generally occurs. Here, I am talking about only very *slight* changes in blood pH.

Which foods are acidic and which are alkaline? Fruits and vegetables are generally alkaline, and most other foods are acidic. The body has a remarkable ability to balance its pH because the proper acid-alkaline balance is critical to health, but when you dump acid into your body, you really put the body at a disadvantage. You need to drink a lot of water just to dilute one can of pop. Soda pop was one of the drinks I always implored patients to remove from their diets if they wanted to regain their health. All sodas, even diet sodas, wreak havoc with the body, making it extremely difficult to attain or even maintain good health. Distilled water is a little on the acidic side, but the cleansing properties of steam-distilled water far outweigh the acidity.

ROOM TEMPERATURE LIQUIDS

I do not drink my liquids cold. If a beverage has been stored in the refrigerator, I take the liquid out of the fridge and wait until it approaches room temperature before drinking it. We all know that the human body's internal temperature is around 98.6°F, although this varies slightly from person to person. When you pour cold liquid into a warm body, you place an added burden on the digestive system because the system has to warm the liquid up before it can start to absorb the beverage's nutrients. You really should drink cool drinks only when you are overheated or are suffering from a fever, and therefore want to cool your body down.

OTHER THOUGHTS ABOUT BEVERAGES

When I was in practice, I realized that all my patients had particular foods and beverages that they enjoyed, and I would work with each of them to help them devise a diet that was both enjoyable and healthful. There really were just a few products that I highly suggested patients stay away from, and they, as you might have guessed, included cow's milk and soda. It is an uphill battle to get well and prevent disease when you put these two beverages in your body.

As I discussed earlier in the book, steam-distilled water and freshly made fruit and vegetable juices are my top beverage suggestions, but I also approve the consumption of limited amounts of teas and coffees, as long as they are decaffeinated, preferably organic, and prepared with pure, clean water.

ALISON—A CASE STUDY

Alison came to my clinic complaining of chronic fatigue. She was an "older" lady but felt she could do things someone half her age could do. After I examined Alison, I asked her if she was a regular meat eater and if so, how she prepared her dinner. She stated that she was a "high protein" kind of gal and needed to keep up her strength. Alison went on to say that meat wasn't much good unless you could see a lot of red, both in the meat and running onto the plate! After I settled my own stomach down, I said, "Alison, I bet you have a parasite in your body from eating all that improperly prepared meat." Now her stomach became upset!

I told Alison that she needed to switch from cow's milk to apple cider, which would be used on her morning cereal. I suggested that she use one cup of apple cider on her cereal, and that for the next five days, she place one teaspoon of raw apple cider vinegar in a cup of water and drink it down. Both of these products would kill any parasites that might be lingering in her body from the undercooked meat. I usually wrote down all my instructions for my patients, or I had my nurse write them down, but Alison said emphatically that there was "no need to write anything down," adding that her mind was "as sharp as a tack."

Well, I guess that tack had been rubbed a bit smooth, because at 2:00 AM the next morning, Alison called me to complain that she was experiencing bad stomach pain. I reviewed our conversation from earlier in the day, and she told me she had cereal before she went to bed that evening, and had dutifully poured one cup of raw apple cider vinegar on her cereal. She also drank one teaspoon of apple cider—just like she was supposed to. Well, that would give anyone a stomachache! Alison had gotten her ciders mixed up, along with the amounts.

I told Alison to blend up a banana until it became a soft pudding, and then dip a spoonful of banana in some peanut butter and eat it. Her tummy was way too acidic and needed something alkaline in it. Most fruits are alkaline, with the exception of blueberries and cranberries, and banana is very easily digested and does an excellent job of "coating" the tummy. The next day, Alison's daughter shared with me that her mother had selective hearing. We joked about that one for a long time, but we weren't laughing at 2:00 AM. By the way, Alison now eats only organic, fully cooked meat a couple of times per week, and has organic apple cider on her cereal. Her chronic fatigue cleared up beautifully.

Earlier in this chapter, I mentioned that organic apple cider makes a healthful beverage. It is interesting that both apple cider and raw apple cider vinegar (along with garlic) can kill many of the worms and other parasites that can end up in the intestinal tract, often as the result of improperly prepared food or unhygienic habits. When my daughter was younger, every time she ate cereal with apple cider on it or drank some cider, she would say, "Die, Mr. Worm!" Incidentally, use only apple cider—not apple cider vinegar—on cereal or as a drink. Apple cider vinegar is very potent and should be taken only one teaspoon at a time.

What about caffeine-containing beverages, such as coffee and tea? Organic coffees and teas are fine, provided that the water with which they are made is clean, as discussed in Chapter 1. Decaffeinated forms of coffee and tea are much healthier for you than the standard caffeine-containing forms. Caffeine can act as an artificial stimulant to the body, thus placing stress on the internal organs, the adrenal glands, in particular.

The adrenal glands are part of the endocrine system. Each of the two glands sits atop one of your two kidneys. One of the jobs of the adrenal glands is to excrete adrenaline into the body to boost energy levels. When you drink caffeinated beverages, the caffeine can act as a toxic stimulant and stress the adrenal glands. Consequently, the adrenal glands function less efficiently and over time, you become constantly tired. You then have to drink more caffeine to stimulate the body, and in turn, the adrenal glands become even more stressed and toxic. It is a vicious cycle. If you walk the road to health by following the suggestions made in this book, you will not feel the need to artificially stimulate your body. Let me add that if you do prepare organic decaffeinated coffee and tea, you should think about using chlorine-free filters. That way, you won't be drinking chlorine!

SALT

Mined salt is an inorganic mineral that will harden the vessels and tissues of the body. Maybe this is why our Creator put salt deep inside the earth so we could not get at it.

If you feel that you need to give your food a saltier taste, use sea salt or, better yet, use kelp. Kelp, a natural food from the sea, is an excellent seasoning for food. Kelp is also very beneficial for people who suffer from hypothyroidism. After the age of forty, a great many women find that the thyroid slows down, and they begin to experience symptoms such as cold feet, weight gain, and a general slowing of the metabolism. Sea salt and kelp also help when you are trying to regulate your cholesterol, which so many people are trying to do these days.

Remember to be a label reader when purchasing packaged foods, as many products contain high amounts of inorganic salt to enhance the flavor. This is not the salt you want to be eating.

HEALTHY OILS AND FATS

I recommend using olive oil for baking and coconut oil for cooking. Olive oil, a product from the olive fruit, contains essential fatty acids that the body needs to lubricate joints and to gently cleanse the internal organs. I suggest using cold-pressed extra virgin olive oil simply because there is less processing involved in its production compared with that of other olive oils. Coconut oil is also a wonderful oil to consume, and one that you will read about throughout this book. Because this oil has the ability to withstand higher cooking temperatures than olive oil, it will not break down under high heat. Extra virgin coconut oil is best for cooking. Sesame, sunflower, flaxseed oil, and butter are also good fats to consume. These foods have a healthy mix of the EPA (eicosapentaenoic acid), essential fatty acids, and cholesterol that the body needs to function optimally.

UNHEALTHY OILS

Avoid soy, canola, corn, palm, safflower, and cottonseed oil, as well as any products that contain hydrogenated and partially hydrogenated trans fats. These oils are not nearly as body-friendly as the previously mentioned oils, and definitely contribute to toxic buildup. Hydrogenated oils and trans fats can lead to the breakdown of the myelin sheath surrounding the nerves, especially the nerves in the brain. Myelin, a coating made primarily of fat, aids in the transmission of nerve impulses in the brain. When the myelin sheath is damaged, proper nerve flow connections are not made. Parkinson's and other neurodegenerative conditions, along with heart problems, are a hallmark of broken-down myelin. *The Journal of Nutrition* concludes that "trans fatty acids in adipose tissue are associated with an increased risk of coronary artery disease."[5] The two most important parts of your body—the ticker (heart) and the thinker (mind)—will be negatively affected by these oils.

The gallbladder, too, has a hard time processing hydrogenated and trans fats. Many people suffer from gallstones as a result of the accumulation of unprocessed fat in the gallbladder. If you want to keep your gallbladder stone-free, use olive oil, as it has a wonderful effect on this organ.

Which foods contain trans fats? You will see hydrogenated fats and trans fats listed on many packaged foods, margarine, and vegetable shortening. That's why I recommend that you avoid margarine, a butter substitute. Margarine is simply not a natural food and will lead to a toxic buildup in the system. I live by the axiom that we should eat what the Creator gave us—not what man has made to replace it. The human body simply cannot process fake food. Remember the TV commercial that stated, "It's not nice to fool Mother Nature"? Don't try to fool your body with pretend food or your health will forsake you.

FOODS, FERTILITY, AND HORMONAL BALANCE

As I mentioned earlier, I do not eat any meats or dairy products unless they are organic, free-range, hormone-free, and antibiotic-free. When animals and animal by-products have been injected with hormones, they pass the unnatural hormones directly to us when we eat the foods. The ingestion of these unnatural hormones is a big reason for infertility problems, early puberty, and the early uncomfortable menopause that so many females and yes, even males, experience today. When men go through their "change of life," it is called andropause. However, the "change of life" doesn't have to be so drastic and miserable, nor does puberty have to begin so early and abruptly in life.

Couples in their reproductive years should be able to conceive and be free from many of the infertility and hormonal problems so common today. The unnatural hormones from the meat and dairy that we consume interfere with our own natural hormones, and can cause all kinds of imbalances within the body. Women can exhibit male characteristics, and men can exhibit female characteristics. The *Endocrine Reviews* reports, "The introduction of hormones into cattle feedlots leads to the exposure of individuals who might otherwise not ever in their lives come in contact with such materials." The article continues, "We have to give very serious consideration to its implications for our subsequent development and growth and possibly reproductive functions."[6] Hormone hamburgers don't contribute to a healthy reproductive system.

Whenever the couples I treated told me about infertility problems, one of my first recommendations was to stay away from hormone-fed meat and dairy products. When the couples avoided hormone-fed products, their hormonal systems began to regain their normal balance. When the patients blended or juiced fruits and vegetables along with the seeds, their bodies even more quickly rebalanced the hormones, enabling them to conceive. Seeds are full of Nature's natural hormones. Maybe that is why our Creator gave us seed-bearing plants.

I often recommended that couples trying to conceive use a small dab (teaspoon) of coconut oil on their bodies as a cream. Coconut oil is wonderful at converting the healthy cholesterol in the oil into DHEA (dehydroepiandrosterone). Sometimes called a "mother" hormone, DHEA helps to regulate many of the other hormones produced in the body, including testosterone and estrogen. This easy protocol can be followed by women and men and can resolve more than just fertility issues. Many men reported to me that their prostate problems were alleviated when they avoided hormone-injected meat and used coconut oil. People should not assume that hormonal problems are the result of getting older.

There were times when I had to prescribe an herb called *chaste tree* to female patients, and an herb called *tribulus* to male patients. These herbs help balance hormones and aid with conception, as well as ease people into menopause and andropause. However, I would always suggest coconut oil as the first option, along with seed-containing produce and clean meat and dairy. These natural approaches are far better than the synthetic hormones people utilize when attempting to increase or balance their body's hormone levels. Too often, there is a long-term price that must be paid when synthetic hormones are used.

JULIE AND TERRY—A CASE STUDY

Julie and Terry were referred to me by another physician. The couple had been unable to have what they wanted more than anything—a baby. Julie and Terry yearned to expand their family and had been trying to conceive for several years, but had so far been unsuccessful. They had spent a lot of money on various testing procedures, all of which determined that there was no reason why they couldn't have a child.

After taking their case history, I suggested that they clean up their diet by eating hormone-free meat and dairy and consuming seed-containing fruits, and that they also use a coconut oil rub. Within six months, Terry reported back to me that his wife, Julie, was pregnant. After years of trying to conceive, they were ecstatic to share their news, and eventually named their bundle of joy after me. I thought it was a great honor, but all I had done was help them balance their hormones.

AVOIDING CANNED FOODS

You have probably already noticed that I recommend buying food that is as fresh as possible. Moreover, I strongly suggest that you avoid all canned foods. The nutrient value of canned food is minimal at best, and a host of toxic preservatives are used to keep the food from spoiling in the can. I don't want all those preservatives in my body!

Canned food also poses a threat through the aluminum content of the can, which can leach into the food. Aluminum that has been absorbed into food has been found in the brain and linked with memory problems. In the *Environmental Review*, an article stated, "Prudent avoidance is recommended of products containing and practices yielding potentially bioavailable quantities of aluminum (e.g., aluminum based antacid compounds, processed foods containing aluminum compounds, or acid foods that are cooked or stored in aluminum utensils or foils)."[7]

There is an old saying, "I can't remember what I was supposed to remember!" Perhaps you are supposed to remember to keep aluminum away from your food.

SWEETENERS

Stay away from processed sugars and artificial sweeteners such as aspartame, as these products are toxic to the body and provide no nutritional value. I recently read an article published in the *Texas Heart Institute Journal* which concluded that there were "profound adverse neurologic, cardiopulmonary, endocrine, and allergic effects of aspartame products."[8] Did I get your attention? Think about this the next time someone you know reaches for that little packet of toxin to put in his morning coffee.

Are any sweeteners healthy? When sweetening drinks or baked goods, pure, unfiltered raw honey is a good choice. In its natural state, honey is full of vitamins, minerals, enzymes, and all the other cofactors that make a complete, nutritious food. Another good choice is turbinado sugar, which is a delicious, minimally processed raw sugar. When baking, carob chocolate made from the carob plant is a wonderful minimally processed product, with its vitamins and minerals still intact. Organic dark chocolate is also tasty and full of antioxidants, the natural substances that inhibit the damage caused by oxidation. All of these products will enable you to enjoy sweets that are not only delicious, but healthy, too.

MAKING HEALTHY SUBSTITUTIONS

As I have stated earlier, it is my goal to impart to you, the reader, a lifestyle change—not to advertise the latest diet pill or supplement. I am a great believer in enjoying food and not depriving yourself of something you love to eat.

Let me explain further. Many of my patients were eating things that were causing a toxic buildup, and thereby inhibiting their body's ability to repair and rebuild. I simply suggested that they substitute "good" ingredients for the "bad" ingredients that made up their diet. For example, I enjoy sweets, provided I get in some exercise and burn up some calories. (You'll learn more about exercise in Chapter 4.) My wife is an excellent cook, and she frequently bakes my favorite food, which is chocolate chip cookies. Let's discuss what types of ingredients she uses in these cookies. She starts with organic whole wheat flour, with all its vitamins and minerals still intact, rather than white, refined, nutritionally poor flour. She then adds organic eggs from free-range chickens, not antibiotic-laden eggs; aluminum-free baking soda; cold-pressed extra virgin olive oil; organic oat bran; raw unfiltered honey (not processed white sugar); and finally, carob chocolate chips (not chocolate that has been stripped of its nutrients). Delicious! I am starting to get hungry now. These chocolate chip cookies are full of vitamins and minerals. Like any cookies, they do have their share of calories, so I don't recommend them as a steady diet. But they make nutritionally sound treats. In contrast, if you looked at the nutrition facts on a package of grocery store cookies, you'd find them full of calories but devoid of nutrients. If I am going to eat a cookie, I may as well get some nutrition out of it!

Patients would routinely ask me for healthy recipes that they could prepare for their families. I simply suggested that they replace whatever ingredients they were currently using with the healthy ingredients I have been mentioning. The dish would turn out very much like the original dish, but much healthier—just like my wife's chocolate chip cookies.

When we get away from non-nutritious foods, we can make great strides in regaining our health. Regaining and maintaining health should not involve arduous sacrifice that makes living miserable. We shouldn't have to deprive ourselves by dieting six days a week, only to be "rewarded" on the seventh day. This is commonly called the "cheat day"—the day on which we can splurge and pollute ourselves in any way we want because we deserve a reward after being faithful to our diet all week long. What kind of life is that? By simply replacing unhealthy ingredients with wholesome ones, your days of deprivation will be over, and you won't need to "cheat" on yourself!

DIETS AND WEIGHT LOSS

I would like to address weight loss for a moment. When I had a practice, many patients asked me if I could recommend a special diet that they could purchase or follow. Certainly, every week, a new diet guru purports to have found the latest secret to melting off pounds in a hurry. You'll hear all sorts of promotions such as: "You'll lose two sizes by the time you have that high school reunion." The truth is, there really is no great secret to safe, sensible weight loss, no matter what the latest diet guru claims. It took some time to put the weight on; therefore, it will take some time to get the weight off. Weight loss is big business, but it is not really all that complicated. You simply need to expend more energy (calories) throughout the day than you take into your body via food or liquid.

How can you burn off more calories than you consume? You can start by engaging in some form of continuous physical activity for at least twenty minutes every day. The other aspect of weight loss is eating foods that are as close to their natural state as possible, and drinking natural juices and clean water. That's it! By eating natural foods, you will satisfy your hunger and will not have cravings for the processed sugars and refined flours that so quickly put on pounds. I generally recommend a one- or two-pound loss per week until you reach a healthy goal for your height and body type.

You probably know that you can lose weight much faster if you follow a drastic diet. We have all heard of the grapefruit juice diet and even the candy bar diet. (Yes, if you just eat two candy bars per day and nothing else, you will lose weight.) What about the high protein-low carbohydrate diet, or the high carbohydrate-low protein diet? There are diets to match your particular personality and diets that depend on the weather and season. Fad diets come and go, but they aren't healthy and they seldom achieve long-term results.

I recently watched a big report on one of the national television networks. Scientists had studied weight loss and had come up with new and important information. Stay tuned! So I stayed tuned, and it turned out that the latest and newest information on weight loss was that to lose weight, you have to eat less. I had to laugh! Who pays for these studies anyway? It is simple math: Burn more calories through exercise than you take in through food, and the pounds will come off.

METABOLISM

Many people drink special shakes or eat special packaged foods designed to melt away the pounds. So often, these "special" shakes and meals are loaded with preservatives and ingredients that you can't even pronounce. Many of these products are made to increase your metabolism, which determines how many calories you burn. But what happens when you stop eating these foods? The metabolism returns to its original level and the pounds go back on.

There is another point that I would like to make. Is it safe to increase the body's metabolism unnaturally? Increasing metabolism is one of the purposes of exercise. The body burns calories not only when you exercise, but also when you are at rest after you have completed the exercise. Exercise is a *natural* way to set your metabolism higher.

CALORIES

A calorie is simply a unit of energy. Besides calories, many packaged diet foods contain toxins such as benzoic acid and a high amount of salt that can accumulate in the body. If your body can't recognize the packaged food ingredients as whole, natural foods, your body will either store the ingredients as toxins or eliminate the foods from the body, giving you no nutritional benefit. Either way, these new diet plans don't sound all that great to me! Our Creator has designed our body to eat a variety of foods as close to their natural state as possible and to increase our metabolism naturally.

Many athletes drink special shakes and eat special muscle-building foods, but whether a man-made food is designed for dieters or athletes, the fact is that these foods cannot be processed by the body. Therefore, the people who use them are loading themselves up with artificial ingredients that the body cannot use or efficiently eliminate.

How many calories can you consume each day to be sure that you take in less than you expend? I don't think your parents and grandparents took out their calculators and punched in caloric formulas to come up with the optimum amount they should consume. They simply lived life! Overall, they followed a much more healthy lifestyle than most people now follow, and they lived for many years. Their bodies reached homeostasis, a natural leveling off, when they were at the optimum weight for their height and body structure. Nature will dictate this for you naturally.

You will intuitively realize that increasing your gentle exercise in duration, maybe up to thirty minutes on some days, will help you attain and maintain your optimum weight. By consuming healthy foods and getting physical activity, you will lose weight the no-stress way. You may find that you have to cut down on snacks between meals, or simply reduce the portions you eat at mealtime, but you won't have to worry about "falling off" a particular diet because you won't be on one. You will be eating as part of an overall natural lifestyle, much as your ancestors did before the influx of processed foods, fast foods, and man-made foods contributed to obesity and other health issues.

BILL—A CASE STUDY

Bill was forty-three years old and had been rather slim for much of his life. He had never really thought much about his weight, but when he turned forty, he noticed that he was starting to put on a few pounds. He wasn't overly concerned, but he did mention it to me when I saw him at my clinic. What initially brought Bill to me was shoulder pain that he experienced after playing softball. I examined his shoulder and diagnosed the problem.

Following Bill's treatment, we discussed his weight. Bill stated that he didn't want his weight to get out of control. He realized that playing softball wasn't going to burn up a ton of calories, so he wanted to do something that would prevent continued weight gain. I shared with Bill that all he need do was start replacing the ingredients in his present diet with healthy ingredients. If he did that, he would have no problem maintaining his weight, and would even lose a few pounds. Bill was relieved because he did not want to embark on the various diets that he saw advertised on TV and in the latest magazines. He also did not want to sacrifice his present lifestyle just so he could have a "cheat day" at the end of each week.

I told Bill that diets simply don't work, and stated that if he started to drink clean water and eat clean foods, with all the nutrients intact, he would be happy with his weight. Bill experienced no mental stress as he took steps to eat better foods. His shoulder healed well and he no longer has weight issues.

SNACKING

If you are like most people, you love to snack between meals. But you generally won't have the desire to snack if your main meals are full of nutrients. The
biggest reason people feel the need to snack—and are hungry so often—is that
their bodies are crying out for nutrition! When the body is being nutritionally
deprived, it demands food.

People ignore the body's cry for nutritionally rich foods. They continually eat to satisfy their hunger, but they don't satisfy their real dietary needs.
I know of people who just "graze" all day long, constantly nibbling and
never really having a meal. This continuous nibbling places stress on the
digestive system because of the body's need to constantly activate digestive
enzymes secreted by the pancreas and hydrochloric acid secreted by the
stomach. Many people who snack often also suffer from heartburn due to the
stomach's continual production of acid. When people graze, the colon (large
intestine) has to serve as a storehouse for all these little snacks until there is
enough waste for the body to excrete. The colon is not designed to be a storehouse for food.

If you do want a between-meals snack, try eating fruit. Fruit is broken down
very quickly in the stomach, giving the digestive system the least amount of
work. The broken-down food, or nutrients, is then absorbed by the small intestine, and the remainder of the food passes into the colon, where it is evacuated
quickly. The longer the food is stored in the colon before evacuation, the more
toxic buildup the body experiences.

CHEWING GUM

Gum chewing is a bad habit for two reasons. The first is something that you
probably realize—your teeth and gums really don't need to be soaked in the
refined sugars or sugar substitutes that ooze out of the gum as you chew. Your
teeth are literally bathed in refined or artificial sugar when you put a stick of
gum in your mouth. Therefore, tooth and gum problems can result.

The second reason gum chewing is harmful is that it stimulates the secretion
of stomach acids and pancreatic enzymes. When you start chewing, the acids are
first secreted by the salivary glands; then the stomach starts readying itself to
digest the food by secreting its own powerful acids, in particular, hydrochloric
acid. The problem is that during gum chewing, there is no actual food for the
acid to digest because you have tricked the body into producing digestive juices.
Then, when a big meal is finally chewed and sent to the stomach, you may find
that you are depleted of your enzymes and acids, and are not able to properly

break down and absorb the food. The result is incomplete digestion, an unhealthy accumulation of food particles in the colon, inadequate nutrition for the body, and improper elimination. When this occurs on a frequent basis, you set yourself up for health problems down the road. Who knew that gum chewing could be so bad?

Taking a Commonsense Approach

Most of us do not have to be on a specific "diet." For the vast majority of people, I suggest a commonsense approach. Should you combine fruits and vegetables together? What about your meat and potatoes? Will peas clash with your corn? What about matching up the colors of the food? Can you imagine what our ancestors would have to say about all this? Good grief! Just eat healthy!

CONCLUSION

You have been given a magnificent body that is designed to use the nutrients provided by real food and excrete the excess organic nutrients that you inadvertently consume. You get into toxic trouble when you consume chemical-laden foods and non-food-based vitamin and mineral supplements, which cause a large amount of inorganic substances to enter the body. The body can't absorb these substances, which then become a burden for the system. By eating a variety of organic, natural foods, your body will extract just the right amount of nutrients for its use and will not be overwhelmed by non-nutrients. (I will talk more about the right kind of supplementation in Chapter 18.)

When your body is free from food-related toxins and has been repaired and rebuilt by nutrient-rich foods, you will no longer crave non-nutritional foods. In addition, by substituting healthful ingredients for unhealthful ingredients, you can still enjoy all your favorite foods. When you do shop for packaged foods, learn to be a label reader. If it isn't natural, you can't pronounce the ingredient, or you don't know what the ingredient is, you probably should avoid the food.

I try to eat as much food as possible in its natural state. The more man interferes with food through processing and refinement, the more nutrition is lost. I try to live by the saying, "If it doesn't come from Nature, I am not going to eat it!" I also like what Hippocrates, the father of medicine, had to say: "Let food be thy medicine and medicine be thy food."

Remember, it's not about diet, it's about lifestyle. One very important part of a healthy lifestyle is the nutrition the body needs to detoxify, repair, and rebuild itself. As you have learned, fruits detoxify and veggies repair and rebuild, so if you put these nutritious foods into your body, you will soon be on the road to alleviating the disorders that plague so many people today. You have just completed the second step on the road to fantastic health.

Remember, Health is Wealth!

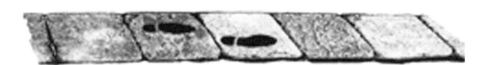

3. Fasting

You deserve a real break today.

When I grew up, I was told to eat my three meals a day, seven days a week. If I didn't eat them, I wouldn't grow up to be big and strong. We are always telling our children to eat, eat, eat! Is it any wonder that the children in our society are experiencing obesity in epidemic proportions?

Despite our country's emphasis on eating, some people do fast on a regular basis. Why? This chapter explores the benefits of fasting and guides you through a health-promoting weekly routine.

WHAT IS FASTING?

Fasting is simply abstaining from food for a period of time—generally, for at least twenty-four hours. There are many people who routinely fast for thirty-six hours or more, and some fast for as long as a week. I sometimes recommend a supervised fast of up to three days or even a week if someone is very sick. But most of the time, a twenty-four-hour fast is good enough for the vast majority of people—including me. On the first day, you eat breakfast, lunch, and dinner as usual, and you begin fasting *after* dinner. The next day, you skip breakfast and lunch, and begin eating again at dinnertime. You may get slightly hungry, but by fasting from the end of one dinner to the start of the next, you will comfortably sleep through the first part of the fast. The next day, you will be able to take your mind off your hunger by keeping yourself busy.

Fasting is not an easy thing to do. It's tough to give up two meals a week when you are so conditioned to having meals—plus snacks!—at regular times of the day. You will probably get hungry and consider fasting for only half the time or perhaps eighteen hours, but if you can stick it out for the twenty-four hours, your health will be all the better for it.

WHY FAST?

In earlier chapters, I explained that many people succumb to ill health because they eat toxin-laden food and—due to an insufficient amount of the clean water needed to flush these poisons out—the toxins accumulate in their bodies. On top of this, many people don't consume the good, clean foods needed to repair and rebuild their health. The result is a body that is stressed as it tries to rid itself of toxins without having the resources it needs to perform this task. This stress leads to ill health.

By helping to eliminate toxins, fasting works towards relieving the stress placed on the body. In fact, fasting may well be one of man's oldest healing agents and has been used for hundreds of years to aid the sick. Fasting is a great internal cleanser. There are a lot of herbs, supplements, and special cleansing programs in the marketplace that claim to clean your internal organs. There are special liver cleanses, kidney cleanses, gallbladder cleanses, and colon cleanses. While many of these are fine, I have found that simple fasting is more effective. Why not perform a whole body cleanse rather than treating only one organ? Also, unlike special products, fasting doesn't cost you anything. In fact, you will actually save money on groceries by skipping meals.

Fasting also provides much-needed rest to the internal organs, especially those involved in digestion and elimination. You probably know that it is important to rest your muscles after exercising. Well, it is also important to allow your internal organs to rest. This gives the body a chance to repair and rebuild.

Many of the longest lived and healthiest people in the world use a regular fasting program to help them achieve excellent health. An article in the *American Journal of Clinical Nutrition* suggests, "Findings to date from both human and animal experiments indicate that alternate day fasting may effectively decrease the risk of cardiovascular disease, whereas results from animal studies suggest a protective effect on cancer risk."[1] While you may not want to fast every other day, I think you'll find that a once-a-week fast can provide great benefits.

Have you ever seen someone who looked radiant—whose skin was so fresh and glowing that it seemed to shine? Fasting is a great way to help the body achieve such a glow because it cleanses all of the organs, including your largest organ, the skin. When I was in private practice and my patients complained of acne, I routinely recommended that they begin a once-a-week fasting program. Their skin problems would soon begin to clear up.

I recommend that children start a regular fasting program when they reach puberty or slightly older, around the age of thirteen. By that time, toxins have started to accumulate in the body. Fasting is especially important when kids have not had the opportunity to eat organic foods and drink clean water.

When Rebecca visited my clinic, she was upset about a severe case of acne and about being slightly overweight for her height and bone structure. I recommended that she eat clean foods and drink clean, pure water, and that she fast once a week. She said that as a teenager, she sometimes found it difficult to get proper food. Her school served breakfast and lunch, but the meals were fried and greasy. I told Rebecca, "Do what you can do." Because Rebecca was determined to feel and look better, she decided to eat breakfast at home and bring lunch and a bottle of water to school. Although she had never heard of fasting, she said she would give it a try.

Three months later, Rebecca returned to the clinic, overjoyed by the results of her efforts. Her acne and weight problems were no longer an issue, and she no longer felt like an awkward teenager. She was more outgoing and felt truly happy.

Rebecca had not been seriously ill when she first came to me, but her weight and skin problems could be seen as symptoms of the unhealthy path she was taking. Because she was willing to adopt healthy habits—not some "quick fix" that would merely cover up her symptoms—Rebecca was able to get the results she was look- ing for and, just as important, to avoid more serious health disorders in the future.

FASTING AND LIQUIDS

During your twenty-four-hour fast, you should consume nothing but clean, pure water with a dash of fresh-squeezed lemon juice. The water-and-lemon juice combination has a powerful cleansing effect, helping the body flush the toxins out of the tissues and eliminate them as waste products.

I do not recommend drinking juices during the fast. If you were to drink store-bought juices, you would actually introduce more toxins into your body because of the additives used to prolong the product's shelf life. If you were to drink home-made all-natural fruit and vegetable juices, despite their liquid form, the body would have to process the juices' nutrients, diminishing the benefits of the fast. However, if you become so hungry that fasting turns into drudgery, it would be better to try a juice fast than to skip fasting altogether. Be sure to make the juice yourself, though, so that the beverage is fresh and absolutely natural. Watermelon juice is a good choice because it is made up mostly of water and, therefore, requires the least amount of digestion. After a few weeks of following a weekly twenty-four-hour fruit juice fast, you may have more success using a lemon water fast.

FASTING WITH DIABETES

If you have diabetes, I suggest that you stir one-half teaspoon of raw honey into the lemon water discussed above. The nutritious honey will help keep your hunger at bay throughout the fast, and at the same time will help keep your blood sugar stable. You may even want to try blended watermelon, seeds included, because of the stabilizing effect of the fiber. Another option is to grind up fruits such as bananas, apples, or pears in a blender, making a fruit smoothie. This high-fiber juice diet will provide at least a partial rest and detoxification for your body. If you have any questions about whether this fast regimen is suitable for you, by all means check with your healthcare provider.

FASTING WHEN ILL

During an acute illness such as the common cold or flu, the body should not be forced to use its healing energy to process snacks and meals. That's why as soon as you come down with an infection, you should stick to a lemon water fast. This will help the body cleanse itself from both accumulated toxins and any harmful bacteria and viruses.

When your body is fighting a viral infection—which usually has symptoms such as a dry cough, clear mucus (if any), and fever—you may want to add a crushed clove of garlic, a teaspoon of raw apple cider vinegar, or one-fourth teaspoon of bee propolis to your lemon water. When taken twice a day, this mixture will help kill the invading virus. A teaspoon of raw honey can be added to make the drink more palatable.

Humbled With Fasting

Psalms 35:13 states, "Yet when they were ill, I put on sackcloth and humbled myself with fasting." (New International Version Holy Bible.) Let me paraphrase this and say, "When you are ill, humble yourself with fasting."

If you are suffering from a bacterial infection—with symptoms such as a phlegm-producing cough, cloudy mucus, and no fever—I suggest that you take one-fourth teaspoon probiotics (such as acidophilus) in capsule, liquid, or powder form; or that you eat a teaspoon of sauerkraut, goat milk kefir (a fermented milk drink), or goat milk yogurt twice a day. By rebuilding your supply of "good" bacteria, these products will enable your body to more quickly and successfully fight the infection.

FASTING SYMPTOMS

When on a fast of any type, you may, of course, feel hungry, and may also experience a headache or mild diarrhea. These are normal reactions. The headache and diarrhea indicate that toxins are being released by the body and are soon to be eliminated as waste. This is the goal of fasting—to get rid of the harmful toxins that burden the body. I have personally never experienced any of these symptoms when fasting; however, some patients have reported them to me. Nevertheless, the vast majority of my patients felt much better after the fast than they had before beginning it.

KAYLA—A CASE STUDY

One afternoon, Kayla entered my clinic in tears. Her high school prom was taking place the next evening and she was feeling sick. She said that the day before, some "sick" kids had coughed on her during a basketball game. She was experiencing a fever of 100°F and had a dry hacking cough.

After treating Kayla, I recommended that she immediately follow a lemon water fast and that she add a clove of raw garlic to each drink. I further suggested a cool bath followed by bed rest. She was advised to repeat the procedure in the evening.

I know that people get very concerned when they or a loved one experiences a fever. Nature has given us this built-in protective mechanism to actually "cook" the offending virus or bacteria, so fevers should cause alarm only when they rise above 103°F or higher. At that point, the high internal body temperature can actually start killing off our healthy cells. When patients are experiencing a fever of 101°F to102°F, I suggest using a room-temperature enema to cool down the body. (For more on this, see page 211 of Chapter 20.) Although Kayla's temperature of 100°F was not a cause for immediate concern, I like to have a few degrees as a safety net. The cool baths and lemon water-and-garlic fast would naturally bring down the young girl's temperature.

Two days later, Kayla called the clinic to say that she was feeling much better and had enjoyed a lovely time at her prom. She told us she felt like Cinderella. I hope that didn't make me the fairy godfather!

ENDING A FAST

Once you have fasted for twenty-four hours, it is important to end the fast by eating either a vegetable or a fruit. A vegetable salad is an especially good choice. This is another reason I like to fast from dinner to dinner: I can break my fast by enjoying a salad. (The thought of a breakfast salad isn't very appealing.)

When you eat salad or uncooked vegetables in their natural state, the food works much like a broom in the intestinal tract. During the fast, the body cleanses itself by dislodging and flushing out many of the toxins in our system. The broom action of the vegetable's "roughage" (fiber) sweeps the colon and actually picks up any residual toxic waste so that it can be excreted from the body. Vegetables are superior to fruits in this respect, but even fruits are better than meats, grains, dairy, and sweets, which should never be your first food after a fast. I would not drink a fruit or vegetable juice right after a fast because roughage is important at this point. After breaking the fast with raw vegetables or fruits, you can continue your meal by eating meats, dairy, grains, seeds, nuts, legumes, sweets, and oils if you so choose.

TONGUE CLEANING

Let me add one last thought about fasting. Since this process releases much of the toxic buildup in the body, it is a good idea to brush or scrape your tongue during a fast. While this sounds silly, the fact is that the tongue is normally full of bacteria, and when you fast, toxins are released from the tongue and mouth. It is beneficial to remove these substances from your body.

To clean your tongue, take a spoon and turn it rounded side up. Then gently scrape the top of your tongue, dragging the spoon from the back of your tongue to the front. Each time you drag the spoon to the front, wash off the spoon under running water. Re-scrape and wash the spoon again. Do this about three times. I think you'll find it a great way to keep your breath and the inside of your mouth feeling clean and fresh.

CONCLUSION

Fasting has been around for many years and has proven beneficial to countless people. If you can incorporate the simple routine of a twenty-four-hour fast into each week, I am confident that you will take yet another step toward attaining and maintaining excellent health. Remember that the purpose of the fast is to release and flush out toxins from the body, and give the internal organs the rest they need to repair and rebuild. Much as the body as a whole needs rest, so do the internal organs—especially, the systems of digestion and elimination. You have now completed your third step on the road to ultimate health.

Remember, Health is Wealth!

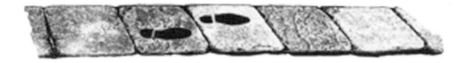

4. Movement and Exercise

How to keep moving
for health and well-being.

When I first began my healthcare practice, after a long day of treating patients, the last thing I wanted to do was exercise. It was also the last thing I wanted to do the following morning. My warm bed was just too comfortable. But once I started a daily exercise routine, I never regretted it because I felt so much better than I had before.

Many years ago, people never thought about exercise regimens because physical movement was part of their daily lives. Our grandparents and great-grandparents did physical work on farms, or walked through village or city streets to get to their jobs. Women had to walk to the market to buy food and other essentials. (Did you ever hear the stories of how your great-grandparents used to walk a mile up a steep hill both to and from school in the snow, barefoot, and in a headwind?)

Modern life is very different, of course. Many of us consider exercise a walk to and from the refrigerator. But it doesn't have to be this way. This chapter will first review the benefits of exercise, and then talk about the many simple steps you can take to get your body moving towards health.

THE BENEFITS OF EXERCISE

Earlier in the book, I stated that the primary cause of sickness is the accumulation of toxins in the body, followed by the body's diminished ability to flush out the toxins and repair and rebuild tissues. Exercise helps the body reverse its disease state and maintain health in several ways. As the result of the stronger flow of blood that occurs during physical activity, fresh oxygen helps the tissues release toxins. These toxins are then moved out of the body through perspiration, excretion, exhalation, and stimulation of the lymphatic system. By working the bones and muscles—including that special muscle known as the heart—exercise also enhances the repairing and rebuilding processes, making the body stronger so that it can better meet the daily demands we place upon it. According to the American Heart Association, "Physical activity or fitness clearly reduces the risk of cardiovascular disease."[1] So in addition to making your visible muscles (the skeletal muscles) more toned and fit, exercise strengthens the body's internal muscles (the smooth muscles) and the cardiac muscle (involuntary striated muscle).

Exactly how many body systems does exercise improve? Exercise:

❑ Enhances the cardiovascular system by strengthening the heart and increasing blood flow in the arteries, veins, and capillaries.

❑ Has a calming effect on the nervous system.

❑ Enhances the respiratory system by strengthening the lungs.

❑ Improves the musculoskeletal system by building strong muscles and bones.

❑ Helps the integumentary system by cleansing the skin.

❑ Enhances the digestive and elimination systems by helping the body break down food and eliminate waste products.

❑ Helps the genitourinary system by strengthening the muscles of the reproductive area.

❑ Enhances the immune system by helping move lymph through the lymphatic ducts.

❑ Helps the endocrine system maintain the hormone levels needed by the body.

In short, exercise benefits the entire body—both the parts you can see and the parts that you can't see, but that nevertheless have a profound effect on your health.

WHAT IS THE BEST EXERCISE?

I have often been asked, "What is the best type of exercise?" Other questions that routinely follow are, "How long should I exercise?" and "How often should I exercise?" Then there's my favorite question, "What is the easiest and least amount of exercise that I have to do?" Remember that I am trying to help you create a healthy lifestyle, one that you will enjoy for the rest of your life. I certainly don't want to give you a boot-camp style of exercise that causes you to agonize as you attempt to melt off pounds in a couple of weeks or months, only to regain the weight when boot camp is over. My goal isn't to make exercising an unpleasant chore.

I see people trying to get "in shape" by lifting heavy weights and playing contact sports such as football and rugby. Now don't get me wrong, these activities are okay. But remember that we are trying to flush out toxins and rebuild tissues. Our goal is health, not brute strength. While there are many exercises to choose from, I recommend those activities that are low on the injury occurrence list because I want you to keep on exercising on a regular basis, and not spend your time recovering from injuries. I generally do not advise sports in which collisions and concussions can, and routinely do, occur. I was once offered free tickets for a weekend of downhill snow skiing. I had never skied before and at the age of forty, the thought of hitting a tree and doing harm not only to myself, but also to the tree, was not appealing. Consequently, a friend took my place and ran into the tree for me. I saw him in my clinic for a treatment the following week! I asked him how the tree fared, but he was not amused.

If you participate in either a contact sport or an activity such as skiing or snowboarding, please take all the proper precautions and consider the exercises discussed in this chapter along with, or in place of, some of the activities in which you now participate. At the risk of sounding like my grandfather, it's important to remind you that you will be older one day, and having a healthy body, unimpaired by years of abuse, will make your later years that much healthier and happier.

Looking at Legs

When I was in practice, I learned I could tell a lot about a patient by looking at the hair on his legs. A lack of leg hair—which is especially common among the senior male population—is often an early indication of problems with the circulatory and cardiovascular systems. When the legs are not supplied with enough oxygen, the body is unable to grow new hair, so when the old hair falls out, it is not replaced. How can you keep oxygen flowing to your legs and other parts of your body? Perform simple aerobic exercise like walking, and your body will get all the oxygen you need.

AEROBIC AND ANAEROBIC EXERCISE

Exercise can loosely be divided into two types—aerobic and anaerobic. Each of these has its own benefits.

Any sustained, rhythmic exercise that is performed for more than one minute is generally classified as being *aerobic*—literally, "with oxygen." Examples of aerobic exercise include brisk walking, running, and swimming. In each of these pursuits, the body is forced to send more oxygen to the muscles in order to complete the activity. As a result, the cardiovascular system becomes stronger and healthier.

An *anaerobic* ("without oxygen") exercise is performed for less than one minute and demands very little increase in oxygen from the body. This type of exercise, which includes short-duration activities such as sprinting and weightlifting, does little to improve cardiovascular function, but does build muscle and bone strength.

Both aerobic and anaerobic exercises are needed for health. In the next few pages, I will describe some of the most beneficial and efficient ways to incorporate these activities into your exercise routine.

Aerobic Exercises

Aerobic exercise improves cardiovascular function and, in doing so, enhances the flow of blood and pumps life-giving oxygen into the body. Best of all, this form of exercise can be as simple and pleasurable as taking a walk.

Walking

Walking is considered an aerobic exercise as long as it is of moderate to high intensity. This means that ideally, when walking, your heart rate should be a little faster than usual, but you should still be able to carry on a conversation. (To learn more about exercise pace, see the inset "Checking Your Pulse During Exercise" on page 72.)

Walking is one of the best forms of exercise you can perform and can be enjoyed by most people. Humans were made to walk. Throughout the centuries, walking was a part of most people's daily routines. The rhythmic activity of arms and legs gently stimulates the lymphatic system, promoting the removal of toxins from the body. Walking also helps strengthen the immune system by circulating germ-fighting white blood cells via the lymphatic fluid, and strengthens and tones the various muscles of the body. It also stimulates the excretion process. If you ever suffer from constipation, a good walk may be all that is required to get your bowels moving properly again. Finally, walking circulates fresh oxygen so that it can flush out any carbon dioxide waste that has accumulated in the body.

I routinely advised my patients to walk, and the results were incredible. My patients felt stronger, had less aches and pains, and enjoyed a feeling of greater well-being, not only physically, but also mentally, socially, emotionally, and yes, even spiritually.

If you make walking part of your exercise routine, I strongly suggest that you vary distance covered and terrain (flat or hilly) rather than always covering the same ground. The alteration of distance, terrain, and (possibly) duration will keep you from experiencing boredom and prevent your body from plateauing. (To learn about plateauing, see the discussion on page 67.)

KARI—A CASE STUDY

Kari came to my clinic because of low back pain. She was a middle-aged mom who had three kids in school and worked at a full-time job. Upon completing my examination of Kari, I concluded that there was nothing wrong with her back except some general weakening of the lower back muscles, which could be cured by a little exercise. As we spoke, Kari said that although she knew that she needed an exercise program, she didn't like to exercise. She had participated in various forms of exercise before, but either became bored or just couldn't find the time to fit it into her day. She had also purchased many of the exercise gadgets shown on television only to try them once and be done with them. She said they made good clothes hangers, though!

I recommended that Kari begin a daily walking program, just a few minutes a day to start, but gradually building up to twenty minutes. I advised a gentle walk first thing in the morning and explained that this was what I did before going to my clinic. This routine would allow Kari to fit in her exercise before her day got too busy.

After just two weeks of daily walking, Kari reported that she felt better not only physically, but also mentally, emotionally, socially, and spiritually. She enjoyed the flexibility that a walking program provided, and appreciated being able to spend some time alone with her thoughts while she was exercising. She also liked the fact that if she chose, she could turn walking into a social activity by including friends and family. In time, Kari's back felt better, and she has kept up her daily walking routine on a consistent basis ever since.

Swimming and Other Water Exercise

Swimming and other types of water exercise, such as deep-water running and shallow-water walking, are wonderful aerobic activities as long as you continue them for several minutes at a time. The supportive nature of the water makes water exercise perfect for people with joint discomfort. And because this is an aerobic activity, it enhances the transport of oxygen to all areas of the body and strengthens the cardiovascular system.

As discussed in Chapter 1, it's important to choose a non-chlorinated pool for your water exercise because chlorine is toxic to the body. If you have a backyard pool, I suggest installing a counter-current swimming pool device in which a stream of water allows you to swim in place. You will be able to continue your swimming without making all those turns! If you do not have your own pool, you may want to consider installing a counter-current pool in your home. If you do not own a pool and cannot have one installed, seek out a health club, gym, or local "Y" that has a non-chlorinated or reduced-chlorinated pool.

Polar Bears and Shrinkage

I happened to see a television documentary that talked about the polar bear and how its private parts are shrinking due to the chlorine and other man-made toxins that have shown up in its swimming waters. While it's true that I probably need a greater variety of channels to watch, it did make me think that the next time I see a chlorinated pool, I may just skip swimming.

Anaerobic Exercises

As you know by now, I advise that everyone partake in some type of whole-body aerobic exercise program. Walking, swimming, and other forms of rhythmic aerobic exercise are probably the most healthful forms of physical activity. However, it is also important to include anaerobic exercises that help strengthen the body. Included among these are body-weight resistance exercises. An article in *The Journal of Nutrition* reported, "Resistance training has a positive effect on multiple risk factors for osteoporotic fractures in previously sedentary postmenopausal women." The article continued, "In a population of 100 nursing home residents, a randomly assigned high intensity strength training program resulted in significant gains in strength and functional status."[2] It has been my experience that even low-intensity strength training programs yield excellent results. And I suggest that you don't wait until you are in a nursing home to begin your strength-building exercise program!

Instead of weight-machine exercises, I prefer body-weight exercises—exercises that use the weight of your own body to build your strength. Weight-machine exercises affect only those muscles that the machine allows you to work. Body-weight exercises involve more muscles because the body must recruit the adjoining muscles to act as stabilizers while you are working a particular muscle or group of muscles. This maximizes your workout time and helps tone both the external (skeletal) muscles that you can see, and the internal (smooth) muscles that make your internal organs function more efficiently. The use of barbells and hand weights can also be effective.

Body-Weight Exercises

At this point, you may be wondering what kinds of body-weight exercises you should use. Let me mention a few that I have found helpful.

Stand with your feet a shoulder width apart and hold your arms out in front of you, parallel to the floor. Take a deep breath through your nose and perform a squatting motion, as if you are going to sit in a chair. Then exhale through pursed lips as you stand up again. This is a great exercise for strengthening the muscles and joints of the knees, hips, buttocks, and lower back.

For the next exercise, stand on the balls of your feet and perform toe-raises by going up and down on your toes, rocking back slightly on your heels each time they are lowered to the floor. This is a great exercise for strengthening the ankles and lower leg muscles.

To strengthen your stomach muscles, lie on your back with your knees bent and your arms crossed over your chest, so that your right hand touches your left shoulder and your left hand touches your right shoulder. Then curl your torso upwards towards your knees, exhaling through the mouth as you move upwards. Take a deep breath through your nose as you lower your torso back to the floor. Your body will allow you to move only a few inches off the ground, but you will really feel your stomach muscles tightening. Your spine will be completely supported by the floor, and there will be no chance of injury to your back or your neck. You are almost done! I feel like I am in an infomercial cheering you on.

For the next exercise, roll onto your stomach, place your palms flat on the floor, and perform an old-fashioned push-up. If a traditional push-up is a bit too challenging, support yourself on your knees rather than your feet, and perform the push-up in this modified position. Be sure to exhale through your mouth as you push yourself up and away from the floor, and take a deep breath through your nose as you lower yourself back to the floor. This exercise is a great way to tone the chest, arms, and shoulders.

The next exercise, called the door pull-up, targets the back muscles. Simply straddle a partially opened door, such as the door to your bedroom, and grab the left-hand doorknob with your left hand, and the right-hand doorknob with your right hand. With your legs slightly bent, lean backwards while holding onto the doorknobs. Then pull yourself back up to the door so that your nose is just a few inches away from the edge. Inhale through your nose as you lean back, and exhale through your mouth as you pull yourself up again. If you want to make the exercise a bit more challenging, wrap a towel around each doorknob and perform the movement while holding the ends of the towel rather than the doorknobs.

For the final exercise, called the press-up, while standing, raise the palms of your hands upwards, pressing them towards the ceiling while you exhale through your mouth. Then lower your arms to shoulder level as you inhale through your nose. This exercise expands the rib cage and improves posture.

The exercises described above will tone your chest, back, shoulders, arms, stomach, legs, and calves. Along the way, they will improve postural and spinal support. In fact, this routine will work both the internal and external muscles of the body either directly or indirectly, and thus help your body perform all of your daily tasks.

By combining body-weight exercises with aerobic activities, clean water, clean food, and fasting, you will place yourself not only on the road to achieving weight-loss goals (if weight loss is an issue for you), but also on the road to overall health. You will help your body avoid the muscle deterioration that often accompanies the natural aging process and will be able to remain independent for many more years. You will also save a lot of money on fancy exercise equipment and gym memberships.

I recommend body-weight exercises for everyone, even the experienced athlete. Athletes can use the body-weight exercises to warm up before they begin lifting weights. Nonathletes can follow the body-weight routine after they walk or perform another type of rhythmic exercise.

Duration, Frequency, and Modification of Body-Weight Exercises

I suggest that each time you do body-weight exercises, you perform ten repetitions of each exercise—first ten reps of the squats, then ten reps of the toe-raises, etc. When you get stronger, if you wish, you can add more repetitions of each exercise to your routine. Perform the exercises every other day, no more than three times per week, to allow adequate recovery of your muscles.

As your muscles become stronger, you can further adapt your body-weight routine by substituting more difficult exercises or by modifying the existing exercises to make them more demanding. For example, instead of the squatting exercise, you can step up and down from a small box or step. This will strengthen the leg muscles through a different challenge. When doing toe-raises, try positioning your toes on the end of a book so they are higher than your heels. When performing push-ups, place your hands upon a box or chair that is either higher or lower than your legs so that you make different demands on your chest, shoulders, arms, and stabilizers.

Another option is to modify the number of repetitions to achieve different goals. If your objective is to build strength in a particular muscle or muscle group, the optimal number of repetitions should be lower—two to eight reps per exercise. If your goal is to build endurance in a particular muscle or muscle group, perform twelve or more repetitions of each exercise. If you want to achieve a balance of strength and endurance, keep your repetitions in the nine to eleven range.

JESSE—A CASE STUDY

Jesse had been a construction worker since his graduation from high school, and he played as hard as he worked. When he came to my clinic, Jesse was having neck problems that he attributed to wearing a hardhat. "No more hardhat for me," said Jesse. He was also concerned that his body might not hold up until he was able to retire from the construction industry.

I examined Jesse and treated his neck. Then I told him that he needed to start taking better care of his body. I shared with Jesse my simple exercise program of walking and body-weight exercise, and discussed the benefits of eating clean food, drinking clean water, and routinely fasting. Jesse decided to incorporate my suggestions into his lifestyle. He was serious about wanting to reach retirement age.

About a month later, I saw Jesse again and he said that he was feeling good. He was doing so well, in fact, that he had told all his construction buddies how they, too, could enjoy a healthier lifestyle. Soon, some of his buddies started coming to my clinic for advice. Now if I could only get Jesse to wear his hardhat again!

Weightlifting

Although body-weight exercises are one of the healthiest forms of anaerobic activity, *light* weightlifting can be good exercise, as well. Light weightlifting has a toning effect on the body and can do a moderate job of eliminating toxins— although not as good a job as aerobic activity.

Some weightlifters perform set after set of lifting exercises. For instance, they will perform a ten-repetition set, take a short rest, do another ten-repetition set, and so on, working again and again on the same muscle group. They perform these multiple sets because they feel that more is better, but this overtrains the muscle group and is therefore not needed.

Instead of performing multiple sets of the same exercise, increase the poundage of the weight being lifted and perform just one set of repetitions on that muscle. Better yet, "warm-up" the muscle being targeted by performing a lighter-weight set of the specific exercise, and then increase the weight for your desired set, performing it at your greatest intensity effort. This is much more efficient in terms of building strength and hastening recovery after the exercise

Exercising Your Eyes

Just as exercising your body can strengthen muscles and improve your health, exercising your eyes can strengthen eye muscles and enhance your vision. Eye exercises are great for children who are faced with the prospect of having to wear eyeglasses for the rest of their lives. But don't think that the following suggestions are just for children; the fact is that these exercises can help people of all ages.

For the first exercise, keep your head still and cover your right eye with your hand. Move the left eye back and forth, up and down, and from one corner of the eye to the other. Repeat this for a total of ten repetitions. Then cover the left eye and repeat the procedure with the right eye. This is a great way to strengthen the eye muscles.

For the next exercise, close your right eye and hold your arm out straight in front of you, with the index finger extended upwards. Use your left eye to look at your index finger, shift your gaze to look at an object that is farther away than your finger, then look back at your index finger again. Repeat this ten times before switching to the other eye. You will notice that first the background behind the finger, then the finger itself, and then again the background will appear out of focus, much as one area of a photo becomes out of focus when you train your camera lens on a different area. This exercise will help strengthen your eyes and enhance your depth perception.

routine. When you return to training, you will be stronger than you were before—not suffering from injuries. A study published in *IronMan* magazine concluded, "Proper training will produce rapid but very steady increases in both strength and muscular mass. . . . Only one set of each exercise was performed in almost all workouts."[3] Often, less is more.

CYCLING YOUR WORKOUTS

If you are an endurance athlete or weightlifter, I highly recommend a yearly "cycling" of your workouts. On week one, during the buildup part of the season, perform your daily workouts at a comfortable pace and intensity for a planned amount of time. On week two, cut back the workload by 25 percent. On week three, equal the workload performed in week one, and on the final week of the month, cut back to 50 percent of your week-one workload. Each month, you should increase the total workload by no more than 10 percent of that of the previous month. When you get closer to the competitive season, switch to a

If you or a family member needs to wear eyeglasses, I suggest that you find a healthcare practitioner who not only prescribes eyeglasses, but also understands eye-correcting exercises. These practitioners will work with you to address the cause of the eye problem and actually improve your vision. Some practitioners strengthen eyes by prescribing lenses that are not the full prescription strength needed to completely correct vision. Although the difference between the full-strength and lesser-strength lenses is imperceptible, the lower strength forces the eye muscles to work harder in order to sharpen the image. This strategy makes the eyes less likely to need stronger prescriptions in the future. The alternative—prescribing full-strength eyeglass lenses—usually necessitates the use of stronger and stronger prescriptions over time because the cause of the problem is being ignored.

A revolutionary form of eyeglasses can also help strengthen the eyes if worn for a few minutes every day. Called *pinhole eyeglasses*, these inexpensive plastic glasses have tiny holes in the lens. When you look through the pinholes, your eyes are forced to converge in a more direct line of sight, cutting down peripheral vision. This is similar to what happens when you squint and reduce your area of vision. The eye focuses and can see very clearly through the pinholes. By retraining the eye, these glasses can eventually enable you to see better even when you are not wearing them.

sport-specific workout routine that will build your strength. Finally, during the competitive season, design your workouts so that they closely match the activity in which you are competing. Once the competitive season has ended, start the cycle over again.

This cycling approach helps relieve burnout and boredom and decreases the chance of injury. For example, if you are a runner, I suggest that you start your early season training by running very easy mileage, remembering the respective workloads as noted above. When you get closer to the start of the competitive season, slightly increase the speed of your running workouts twice a week, and include some hilly terrain to strengthen the sport-specific muscles you will be using during the racing season. When the racing season arrives, continue to increase the speed of your selected workouts—twice a week—with one-mile distances consisting of up-tempo running. Then gradually shorten the distances each week while continuing to increase the speed of the workouts (twice a week) to match the pace of racing you will be doing, leading to the big race at the end of the season.

DEEP BREATHING

When you read about the body-weight exercises on page 61, you learned that it's important to incorporate deep breathing into each exercise. The fact is that controlled deep breathing—performed either during exercise or immediately after it—is an important part of *any* routine because it floods the respiratory system with fresh oxygen, which is picked up by the bloodstream and delivered to all of the cells.

In Chapter 1, I talked about the importance of water and how we can live for only a few days without it. Well, without life-sustaining oxygen, we can live for only a few minutes. Note that in deep, controlled breathing, you breathe in through your nose and out through your mouth for about ten deep breaths. Most people tend to take shallow breaths, but exercise—especially aerobic rhythmic exercise—causes you to breathe more deeply, sending more oxygen to the tissues. This helps the body rid itself of the excess carbon dioxide, a naturally occurring waste product created during respiration.

So the next time you exercise, remember to breathe deeply and fill your body with fresh oxygen. That way, your activity will not only build strong muscle and bone, but also support your respiratory system and eliminate unwanted waste products.

STRETCHING

If exercise is already a part of your life, you are probably accustomed to seeing people "stretch out" their muscles before beginning a physical activity in the belief that they are warming up their bodies so they will not pull a muscle during exercise. Unfortunately, those who stretch out before an activity are actually setting themselves up for an injury rather than preventing one. They are stretching a cold muscle, and we all know that a cold muscle doesn't extend very easily. By forcing this stretch, you can cause micro-tears in your muscles, tendons, and ligaments that can take a long time to heal. The best way to warm up is to begin your planned exercise activity at a very gentle intensity until your muscles feel warm and ready for a more strenuous workout. For example, a runner can warm up by first walking for a few minutes, then change to a slow jog, and gradually move into a run until he reaches the desired workout intensity.

Stretching is, however, a great activity to perform *after* you walk, run, swim, or engage in another exercise. Stretch very gently, avoiding the jerky, bouncing type of stretch that can easily set you up for a pull, tear, strain, or sprain. Take a deep breath through your nose before the stretch, and breathe out slowly and deeply through pursed lips as you relax into the stretch. Hold the position for just a few seconds, performing just one stretch for each muscle group.

The most important stretch of all is that of the lower back, since the lower back muscles tend to tighten up as we get older. Many people, when they first wake up in the morning, immediately think about their lower back to gauge how it feels after several hours of inactivity. Fortunately, there is an easy way to stretch out the back and prepare it for the day's activity.

Lie on your back on the floor, and grab your knees with your hands. While taking in a deep breath, gently pull your knees up toward your stomach and hold them for a few seconds before bringing your legs back down, one leg at a time, as you exhale. Alternatively, you can place both hands on one knee, pull it up to the stomach while inhaling, hold it for a couple of seconds, and exhale while extending the leg out again. Repeat the procedure with the other knee. When I visited a nursing home as a young boy, one of the residents said, "Son, don't ever lose your ability to go down to the floor and get up again." Maybe that's another reason why I am a big floor-exercise advocate.

You can take the stretch a step further by stretching your lower back and the backs of your legs (the hamstring muscles) at the same time. Lie on your back with your right leg straight on the floor in front of you and your left leg bent with the sole of your foot flat on the floor. Using both hands, grab the back of your right leg and, breathing in, raise the leg in the air, trying to get the sole of the right foot to face the ceiling. Hold the stretch for a few seconds, and exhale as you lower it to the ground. Now straighten your left leg, bend your right leg, and repeat the exercise by raising the left leg with your hands. Don't forget to breathe.

By stretching your lower back, you will also keep your hips and pelvis flexible. For excellent results, combine this stretch with the curl-ups discussed on page 61.

Yoga and Pilates

Yoga is an ancient discipline that combines breathing, stretching, and meditation. Pilates combines stretching and strengthening using the individual's body weight. Both, if done correctly, can be beneficial, although they should not replace aerobic activities like walking.

PLATEAUING

The term plateauing is used to describe a leveling-off point where, despite continuing to walk, swim, or otherwise exercise, no apparent improvement is being made. If you do not need to lose weight and you are not training for athletic competition, plateauing is fine. But if it is important for you to reach further levels of fitness or weight loss, you should try varying or increasing the time you spend exercising or increasing the difficulty of the activity. For instance, if walking is your primary form of exercise, I suggest sometimes walking on a level surface, and sometimes walking up a hill or dirt path; sometimes walking briskly, and sometimes using a slow jog. If you generally walk twenty minutes a day, walk for thirty minutes whenever you have the time. These are all great ways to burn more calories and increase fitness while avoiding a plateau.

EXERCISE AND BALANCE

As people age, they tend to lose their sense of balance, which can—and often does—result in falls and other accidents. A simple exercise to help retain balance is to incorporate the one-legged stand for about ten seconds per leg per day. The what? Let me explain. Stand on your right leg for a count of ten, with your left leg lifted up slightly and bent at a 45-degree angle. Now stand on your left leg, bend your right leg, and repeat for a count of ten. If you feel unbalanced during the exercise, steady yourself by holding onto a chair. In time, you won't need to hold onto anything. I usually perform this routine after my walk, body-weight exercises, and stretching. It is a simple and effective way to help retain your balance as you age.

EXERCISE AND HORMONE PRODUCTION

Because of an aging-related decrease in the production of hormones—most notably, testosterone—men and women alike experience diminished endurance, strength, and flexibility as they get older. The body reaches its physical zenith in the early to mid-twenties, after which there is a gradual decline. I know this sounds depressing, but don't be disheartened! Exercise can slow down the aging process so that you can remain vibrant well into old age.

Because hormone production slows down as you get older, many people, including athletes, resort to synthetic (artificial) hormones as a means of finding the fountain of youth. This often results in serious health problems. For a moment, consider how tricky synthetic hormone use can be. How can you determine how much synthetic hormone is needed to replace your natural hormones? And, if you can determine the correct amount, how can your body recognize and utilize the isolated synthetic hormone without developing other health issues?

An article in the *MicroNutra Health Journal* stated, "Synthetic hormones are all organically foreign to the body and are derived from different organisms. Particularly, estrogen used in hormone replacement therapy is derived from the urine of a pregnant mare."[4] Unbelievable! Along with staying away from hormones in pill form, I recommend that you stay away from hormone-laden foods, such as supermarket beef. As discussed in Chapter 2, you should eat fruits and vegetables with the seeds still in them, whole grains, an assortment of nuts and other seeds, healthy oils such as coconut, and limited amounts of meat, fish, and dairy—all of which should be organically raised. This diet will help balance the body's natural hormones, slowing down the loss of strength, endurance, and flexibility.

EXERCISE AND ENJOYMENT

One of the keys to good health is making exercise enjoyable—not something to be dreaded. Remember that during exercise, you can think about your day, pray, or socialize with friends and family. That's a big reason why rhythmic exercise is so good not only for the body, but also for the mind and soul, as well as for emotional and social well-being. After I walk, I feel better in so many ways. It's not just my body that's benefitting from my daily walk.

Walking, swimming, water walking, water running, rollerblading, cross-country skiing, Nordic walking (walking with poles), and jogging are all excellent and enjoyable whole-body rhythmic exercises. If you like to play tennis, bowl, or engage in another sport, by all means continue with those activities. Just incorporate rhythmic whole-body exercises at least three times a week for twenty to thirty minutes, preferably on the days that you aren't involved in your other activities.

Many people have told me that they don't like to exercise because it hurts. If you experience pain while performing any exercise, decrease the intensity or duration of the workout, switch to another type of exercise, or stop the exercise altogether until you feel better. Keep in mind that exercise is not supposed to be painful. If you are experiencing pain in your muscles, this is an indication that you are performing the activity too vigorously or for too long a period of time. Decrease intensity and duration as needed, and build your fitness gradually. If you experience joint pain during exercise, choose a different activity. If knee pain is a recurring problem when walking, be sure to perform the squats discussed on page 61. If you are experiencing joint pain in several areas of the body, I suggest doing an exercise called rebounding. (See page 70.)

If you experience chest pain or shortness of breath during your workout, immediately stop the exercise and resume again on another day, but with greatly decreased intensity and duration. If the pain or shortness of breath does not subside within a few seconds of stopping the activity, or if it starts up again when you resume the activity, call your healthcare provider immediately.

REBOUNDING

Rebounding is gently bouncing up and down on a mini-trampoline. I know it sounds silly, but rebounding does have its health benefits chiefly because it helps circulate the body's fluids—primarily, the lymphatic fluids. This, in turn, helps the body detoxify and strengthens the immune system. Of course, rhythmic exercise such as walking does the best job of circulating fluids, but if you are unable to perform other rhythmic exercise, a few minutes of rebounding is a good alternative. If you enjoy rebounding but are able to walk, I encourage you to engage in walking as your primary exercise and rebound *after* your walk.

BICYCLING

I am not a big proponent of bicycle riding for two reasons. The first reason is the high probability that you will eventually crash. The second reason—and this is just for men—is that the bicycle is not a friend to the prostate gland.

Many men are told to start an exercise program when they develop prostate problems. Bicycle riding is then sometimes suggested. The problem is that the tiny bicycle seat is so narrow that it wedges into the prostate—the little walnut-shaped gland located below the bladder and between the "sit" bones. The man not only has his weight sitting directly upon his prostate when riding, but when going over each and every bump in the road, that little wedge of a seat is slamming into his prostate. The same is true of the wider, softer seats some men use when cycling. Their weight is still directly over their prostate.

Journal Report

An article in *European Urology* stated, "The most common bicycling associated urogenital problems are nerve entrapment syndromes presenting as genital numbness, followed by erectile dysfunction."[5] This kind of information is enough to get me off the bike!

I realize that there are many men who have ridden their bikes for a long time and have experienced no problems, but in practice, I have seen a direct connection between prostate problems and bicycle riding. If you must ride, I highly suggest that you look into buying a bicycle seat that has a pre-cut opening which takes pressure off your prostate. Bicycle seat manufactures are becoming increasingly aware of this necessity. I also suggest that you wear protective gear such as a helmet. Accidents do happen, and when you're on a bicycle—and therefore unprotected as you would be in a car—a helmet can truly be a lifesaver.

ADAM—A CASE STUDY

Adam was a proud father of two very active boys. Adam himself was very ener-getic and liked to participate in many of the sporting activities that his boys enjoyed. One afternoon, this father of two visited my clinic because he was having headaches. During my examination, he began to discuss another health issue that was concerning him. Adam was experiencing soreness in the area underneath and between his legs and was feeling numbness in his genitals. In an effort to lose weight, he had been riding one of his son's bicycles for about thirty minutes every night after work. He wasn't losing weight, and he was feeling pain.

Following treatment for his headaches—which were not related to his other problem—I advised Adam to get off the bicycle and start a walking program. He would lose weight faster than he would riding a bike because more muscles would be involved, and his prostate soreness would go away as well. I called Adam a few days later to check on his headaches and prostate. He said that both problems had cleared up. No more bike riding for Adam.

You may be wondering what is good for the prostate besides clean water, food, fasting, and the exercises recommended earlier in the chapter. Sex! Now that I have your attention, let me clarify. The prostate produces a portion of the fluid that makes up semen, the fluid expelled during sexual activity. A study published by the American Medial Association reported "The prostate accumu-lates carcinogens, which are perhaps cleared out during the male sex act."[6] Sex, therefore, is almost like an oil change. Old fluid is flushed out of the prostate, making way for fresh new fluid. I won't get into how often one should engage in this activity; my point is that the expulsion of old fluid is healthy. Keep in mind, though, that clean water, clean food, fasting, and exercise are far more important not only for prostate health, but for overall well-being.

Exercise and Fasting

In Chapter 3, you learned the health benefits of a twenty-four-hour fast. Can you combine exercise with fasting? Good question! During your twenty-four-hour fast, you should refrain from exercise. If you start your fast on a Saturday night, for example, take a break from exercising on Sunday. Let your body do its job of detoxifying, repairing, and rebuilding during the fast, and you'll soon feel stronger and more fit.

Checking Your Pulse During Exercise

Earlier in the chapter, I mentioned that when walking, you should adopt a pace that permits you to comfortably carry on a conversation. By maintaining a "conversational pace," you can help ensure that your exercise does not place undue stress on your heart. You can also monitor your exercise pace by taking your pulse.

Your pulse is the number of times your heart beats in one minute. To determine it, place the tips of your index, second, and third fingers on the palm side of your other wrist, below the base of the thumb. Press lightly until you feel the blood pulsing. Using a watch or clock with a second hand, count the beats that you feel for ten seconds. Multiply this by six to get your pulse per minute.

Once you know your pulse rate, you can evaluate it to see if it is in a healthy range for your age. First, determine your *maximum heart rate* by subtracting your age from 220. For instance, if you're 30 years of age, your maximum heart rate is 190 (220 - 30 = 190). When you exercise, you want to stay within 60 to 80 percent of your maximum heart rate. This is called your *target heart rate,* and you can determine it simply by multiplying your maximum heart rate first by 60 percent, and then by 80 percent. So if your maximum heart rate is 190, your target zone extends from 114 to 152 beats per minute. (190 x 60% = 114. 190 x 80% = 152.) If your pulse is higher than this when you exercise, you should probably exercise at a slower, less strenuous pace and build your fitness up gradually.

If you have trouble taking your own pulse, you're not alone. A lot of people choose to use heart rate monitors so that pulse taking is easier and more accurate. Available in sports stores, these watch-shaped devices make it simple to check your pulse during physical activity.

CONCLUSION

Lack of physical activity can cause a host of problems, from a weak heart and circulatory system to muscles that are unable to perform daily tasks. Fortunately, these problems and more can be corrected through a program that combines aerobic rhythmic exercise, such as walking, with gentle anaerobic activity, such as body-weight movements, along with flexibility and balance exercises. These exercises will rebuild and repair the body, and help avoid many serious health problems.

Remember to use deep breathing during exercise, and especially, to use deep breathing outdoors. Many people walk on a treadmill during inclement weather, and this is fine, but after using the treadmill, step outside for a minute and breathe in some fresh air. This will enable you to take in more oxygen, which is one of Nature's most potent detoxifiers. Most important, have fun with exercise. You have just completed step four on the road to supreme health.

Remember, Health is Wealth!

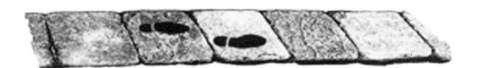

5. Sunlight

Let the sun shine!

The poor sun has been getting a really bad reputation lately. It has been accused of causing a host of skin problems and diseases. We are told to slather on sunscreen, wear wide-brimmed hats, wear sunglasses that wrap around the sides of our heads, put on long-sleeved shirts and long pants, and hope the sun doesn't zap us. Better yet, we should just stay indoors. How come all of a sudden the sun is so harmful?

The truth is that the sun isn't bad. Quite the contrary! The sun is extremely good for you and the risks of staying out of the sun are worse than the so-called risks of being in the sun. Sunlight has incredible health benefits. If there were no sun, I'm afraid we would all die fairly quickly as the life-sustaining plants, animals, and water would disappear from the Earth.

In earlier chapters of this book, I discussed the importance of detoxifying the body. Well, the sun is one of Nature's best known detoxifiers. When you spend time in the sun you tend to perspire, and perspiration eliminates toxins through the skin's pores. The sun, with its perfectly balanced UVA (ultraviolet type A) and UVB (ultraviolet type B) light ray spectrum, is excellent at killing infections that occur in and on your body. Just a few decades ago, many physicians recommended that their patients get a few minutes of sunlight exposure each day to help relieve a myriad of health problems. I always suggested that my patients include more sunlight, not less, in their lives.

VITAMIN D

When the skin is exposed to sunlight, the ultraviolet rays trigger synthesis of vitamin D, which, along with calcium, helps to build strong bones. It is sad for me to see so many people with osteoporosis load up on calcium and other "bone-building" supplements only to have their conditions continually worsen. New patients would come into my clinic and exclaim in horror that for years, they had taken calcium pills and consumed grocery-store milk for the purpose of building up their bones, and now they had arthritis and osteoporosis! The man-made pills and denatured milk were not recognized by the body as food. Therefore, the calcium was not absorbed by the body and utilized to build strong bones. The bones, over time, were actually becoming weaker as a result of not having enough calcium-containing vegetables, eggs, and raw cheese, and not enough sun exposure to make vitamin D.

By spending a moderate amount of time outdoors, as described on page 76 of this chapter, and eating clean fresh foods, as described in Chapter 2, you will get the vitamin D your body needs to attain and maintain excellent bone health.

Journal Report

The *Journal of the National Cancer Institute* published a report stating, "Evidence is beginning to emerge that sunlight exposure, particularly as it relates to vitamin D synthesized in the skin under the influence of solar radiation, might have a beneficial influence for certain cancers."[1] See, I told you the sun was good for you.

DEPRESSION

One way to get on the path of better mental health is to spend some time in the sun. It's worth noting how many people become depressed and lethargic when sunlight is reduced or not present for a period of time. According to an article published by the American Academy of Family Physicians regarding seasonal affective disorder (SAD), "SAD may be related to changes in the amount of daylight we get."[2] While the specific causes of SAD are not known, a strong link has been established between symptoms of depression and reduced natural light. I know that if I don't see the sun for a few days, I get sad.

For those people who live in areas where the sun doesn't shine for months at a time, natural daylight spectrum lighting, sometimes called full-spectrum lighting, is a good option. These special light bulbs simulate the color and ultraviolet spectrum of the sun. Although it can't provide the sun's healing properties, full-spectrum lighting does seem to brighten up people's moods.

SUNLIGHT AND SKIN HEALTH

Have you ever noticed how many seniors have skin that looks starved of color—pale and ashen? If more senior centers would simply wheel their patients out into the sun for a few minutes a day, both their skin color and their overall health would improve.

I routinely suggested that all my wheelchair-bound patients spend some time in the sun each day with their bare feet on the ground, soaking up the energy of the earth. This may sound silly to you, and it did sound silly to many of the patients at first. When they followed my suggestion, however, they reported feeling more vibrant as a result of getting in tune with Nature's frequency. What can be more natural than utilizing the sun and the earth to aid us in achieving good health?

When my patients had skin problems ranging from psoriasis to acne, I suggested that they needed more sun on their skin, not less. The Psoriasis Association published an article that concluded, "Approximately 80 percent of people with psoriasis notice an improvement in their skin after they have been in the sunshine. . . . UV light helps to power chemical reactions that affect the function of skin cells."[3] I would venture to say that if those same people made clean water and food a part of their daily lives, the percentage of improved cases would be even higher!

Exposure to sunlight is an excellent way to attain a vibrant glow, too. Think about fruit that ripens in the sun, developing vital color, or of the rainbow created by the sun's reflective rays. Eating a diet of sun-drenched fresh fruits and vegetables with their assortment of beautiful colors will help your skin radiate good health.

SUN SMARTS

The sun's rays are an excellent healer and detoxifier, but you need to follow some simple guidelines so that you can get maximum benefits.

It is best to take advantage of the sun before 10:00 AM and after 4:00 PM because it is during these periods that you will experience the healing ultraviolet A rays. These rays tend to be absorbed into the body, where they provide a range of overall health benefits. Between 10:00 AM and 4:00 PM , the more intense ultraviolet B rays—which are more likely to cause burning of the skin—shine more directly upon the earth. You will receive both types of ultraviolet rays in the early morning and the late afternoon, but the ratio will be more beneficial.

How long and how often should you spend time in the sun? I suggest that you start with five-minute sessions for a couple of weeks, then progress to six-minute sessions for a couple more weeks, and continue to increase the sessions by one minute every two weeks until you are remaining in the sun for twenty minutes at a time. Ideally, you should strive for two to three sessions a week, but if you can add a couple more days of sunning, that's great. To detoxify, repair, and rebuild the body, a twenty-minute session is really all you need. I usually get twenty minutes of sun daily during my walk. Now, you might be thinking

PAUL—A CASE STUDY

I met Paul, age sixty-five, through his caregiver. She had brought Paul to my clinic hoping that something could be done for him. Paul told me he was sick and tired of feeling sick and tired. He spent most of his days in a wheelchair because he just didn't have the energy to get out of the chair and take care of himself. He didn't suffer from any physical disability. He had quit his job about a year before, and hadn't done much of anything since. His caregiver wasn't too sympathetic to Paul's complaints. I think she had grown tired of hearing them!

I suggested that every day, Paul's caregiver wheel him out onto his lawn, put his bare feet on the grass, and let the sun shine down on him for five minutes. The caregiver was advised to do this for two weeks and then let me know how he was doing. She thought I was crazy, but she did it— and I didn't have to wait two weeks to learn the results. After just one week, she called and told me that Paul was feeling better and was starting to have a vibrancy about him. Eventually, Paul increased his time in the sun to twenty minutes a day.

Paul now spends time outside on most days, absorbing the sun's radiant energy and the Earth's magnetic energy. His wheelchair sits in his garage alongside his old exercise equipment. Now he has two extra coat racks. Paul no longer needs a caregiver, but now and again, she stops by to visit him and join him outside. I don't know if she still thinks I am crazy. (Maybe I am better off leaving that question unanswered.) Paul also gets in a daily walk, and when he finishes his walk, he offers his former caregiver a glass of carrot juice from time to time. Who would have thought it?! After seeing Paul's recovery, she started to implement my suggestions in her own life. In fact, she took it a step further by including a day of fasting in her week and drinking clean water. One day, her husband saw her with a wrench in her hand, unscrewing her shower head to put in a filter. He didn't know what to think, but I did . . . and I thought it was a great idea.

that it's easy to spend five or ten minutes in the sun. After all, you get that much sun just walking to and from your car in the supermarket parking lot. Sorry, but that doesn't count as continual health-benefitting sun exposure. That is like walking to the refrigerator and back to the couch and counting it as part of your daily walk.

You need to spend time in the sun with as little clothing on as possible, depending on your privacy situation. Many men can incorporate some sun in their early morning walk by wearing shorts and no shirt, as I often do. Women can wear shorts and a simple tank top in order to absorb maximum healthy rays. If you have a private "sunning" area and are comfortable wearing even less attire, then by all means, do so. The greater the area of the body exposed to the sun, the more healing rays you will absorb.

The Midday Sun

Did you know that during the middle of the day, the proportion of ultraviolet B rays increases? This is when the sun is at its strongest, and why catching early-morning or late-afternoon sun is advisable.

If you live in the northern latitudes, where it is cold and snows often, I suggest that if you have a porch, you sit comfortably on it for a few minutes a day. An alternative is to open your garage door and sit at an angle that allows the sun to gently warm your skin. The sun's rays need to shine directly on your skin and not come through a window or a screen, because the window or screen will act as a filter. If you have to bundle up so that only your face is exposed to the healing benefits of the sun's rays, that is better than no rays at all. Now, I don't expect you to remain in your garage when temperatures are below zero. However, there are many lovely winter days that will enable you to stay in the sun for several minutes. You can also absorb some of the sun's rays by going for a walk with your face or entire head exposed. I just want to remind you that it is my goal to make the recommendations in this book as easy to incorporate and as practical as possible. Remember my motto: "Do what you can do."

EXCESSIVE SUNLIGHT

Can you overdo the sun? Of course you can, just as you can overdo anything else, including eating, drinking, and even exercise. Spending too much time in the sun can lead to overdrying of the skin and, of course, to sunburn. This is more likely to occur in the middle of the day, when there is a higher proportion of ultraviolet B rays. When the skin burns—even if it just turns pink—the skin rapidly produces new cells to heal the burn. Repeated burning leads to repeated overproduction of new skin cells, which can cause abnormal cells—benign or cancerous—to develop. That's why it's so important to stay out of the midday sun.

What about the golden tan many of us seek? Can't you just rush out and get a beautiful tan during your next two-week vacation—or even over the next sunny weekend? Unfortunately, that is like trying to lose forty pounds in two weeks, or trying to begin training for a marathon that's only two weeks away. You can do it, but it's not healthy for you.

You can, however, get a safe tan by spending time in the sun in the early morning or later afternoon. It will take longer, but good health is well worth the investment of time. A tan is not some unnatural reaction to the sun; it is Nature's built-in protective mechanism to prevent the skin from burning, and it is not harmful if you get it over a longer period of time. Many people who are born with naturally darker skin pigmentation feel that they can spend as much time in the sun as they like at any time of the day. Even darker skin, though, should be tanned gradually and should not be exposed to the midday sun, as burning can easily occur, sometimes without your being aware of it.

Suntanning beds are another thing that should be avoided if you are trying to get a tan healthfully. The rays emitted by a tanning bed are much more intense than natural rays. You simply can't change your skin color that quickly without paying a price in terms of health

If you are adamant about avoiding a tan, I suggest that you absorb some UVA rays for five minutes at a time, a couple of days a week. Some healing sun is a whole lot better than no sun at all.

SUNSCREENS

Many people ask me about sunscreens and sunblocks. These products are different from each other, as you can tell by their names. A *sunscreen* actually absorbs the sun's rays, reducing the amount that can penetrate the skin. *Sunblocks*, on the other hand, act as physical barriers, blocking UVA and UVB radiation from reaching the skin. These products do defeat the purpose of spending time under the sun's healing rays. In addition, they coat the skin with unnatural chemicals that can then be absorbed into the body. Moreover, I believe that they are not necessary if you sun yourself only in the early morning and the late afternoon, as I suggest. If you must be in the midday sun, I suggest that you use a more natural means of protecting your skin. If your exposure to the midday sun is only occasional, cover the exposed areas of your body with light-colored clothing that will reflect the UV rays. If you consistently spend time in the midday sun, add a hat as well.

Many of the skin problems that have recently been reported are due to people rushing out to get their tans in a short period of time, or slathering unnatural chemicals on their bodies and then exposing their skin to the midday sun. An article in the *American Journal of Public Health* stated, "Although sunscreens, including PABA and its esters (such as Padimate O) prevent sunburn, there has never been any epidemiological or laboratory evidence that they prevent either melanoma or basal cell carcinoma in humans. Worldwide, the countries where chemical sunscreens have been recommended and adopted have experienced the greatest rise in cutaneous malignant melanoma, with a contemporaneous rise in death rates."[4] Please consider this the next time you reach for that bottle of commercial sunscreen.

The only time I use protection other than clothing—or wear sunglasses, for that matter—is when I am at the beach or in the snow, and the intense rays are reflecting off the water, sand, or snow. This reflection magnifies the sun's rays, making protection necessary. I then use a sunblock on the areas that are not covered by my clothing. The best type of sunblock, and the only one I use, contains zinc oxide. Another product that's handy—but only *after* sun exposure—is coconut oil. At that point, the oil will help your skin retain its natural oils and remain soft. If you have a sunburn, coconut oil will also help speed the healing process.

ALFRED—A CASE STUDY

Alfred was a senior patient who was brought into my clinic by his home nurse. I had treated him a few years before for an injured hip that he suffered as a result of slipping on a wet floor. Alfred, as I remembered him, was a cheerful guy who always had a big smile on his face and a joke to tell. "Dr. Senne, did you hear the one about . . . ?" But this time, Alfred was not in a smiling mood. He mentioned that his knee was really bothering him due to a tumble he had taken a week earlier, and he was very concerned because it was causing him to limp. In addition, there was a nasty cut on his knee as a result of the fall. His nurse (bless her heart), had done what she thought best and wrapped his knee up, hoping it would get better. Unfortunately the wrap not only reduced his range of motion, but also caused the cut to worsen.

The first thing I did was to remove the wrap and restore the range of motion with a chiropractic adjustment. I then utilized a little acupuncture to help initiate the healing of the cut. When this was done, I told Alfred and his nurse to take care of the cut by removing the bandage every day for five minutes, and exposing the area to the healing rays of the sun. The nurse should then rebandage the wound until bedtime, when the dressing would again be removed so that the cut would be exposed to the air overnight.

As for cleaning the wound, I instructed the nurse to cleanse it every evening with raw apple cider vinegar, which acts as an antiseptic, She would then mix together a little coconut oil, jojoba oil, and raw honey, and apply the healing balm to the cut. There is a saying, "If it is good enough to be put on the body, then it should be good enough to be put in the body." For the most part, this holds true because what we put on our skin does get absorbed into the body.

I called Alfred one week later, and he told me that his skin was completely healed. He was even going to start a walking program on the days he didn't dance. When I said I didn't know he danced, he replied that with his knee feeling so good, he was going to start taking lessons.

THE BEST USE OF SUNGLASSES

Earlier in the chapter, I mentioned that I wear sunglasses only when I spend time at the beach or in the snow, both of which magnify the sun's rays through reflection so that protection is a necessity. At these times, a pair of sunglasses enables me to see my surroundings without discomfort and also protects my eyes from the sun's rays.

Many people, however, put on sunglasses whenever they step outdoors, and some even wear them indoors. I try to discourage people from wearing sunglasses when the level of outdoor light is comfortable, and especially when indoors. The eyes were made to absorb light, and when constantly subjected to a dark or dim environment, they adapt to their surroundings and become less efficient at utilizing their light and color receptors (rods and cones). The old saying "Use it or lose it" applies to the eyes just as it does to so many other body structures. We have all seen movies in which a character was kept in solitary confinement with no light for an extended period of time. When the person finally emerged from the darkness, it took some time before his eyes adjusted to the light. I would venture to say that in a situation such as this, not all the rods and cones would ever regain full capacity with regard to light absorption and color reception, depending on how long the individual was kept in darkness. Your eyes need to be exposed to sunlight in order to stay in good working order.

Some people wear their sunglasses during the day to prevent sun-related headaches. If you are prone to getting headaches in the sun, I suggest "sunning" your eyes, as explained in the sidebar below. This will safely condition your eyes to sunlight so that you will eventually be more comfortable and better able to see on a sunny day without strain.

Sunning the Eyes

In my practice, I would encourage patients to "sun" their eyes. To do this, you simply look in the direction of the sun with your *eyes closed*, and gently turn your head back and forth almost as if your eyes were drinking in the sun's rays. During this process, your eyes will feel full of light, as if you were shining a lamp all the way to the backs of the eyes. When you open your eyes again, your vision will be enhanced. Just remember that you should never stare into the sun. Safe sunning of the eyes is performed with your eyes closed, not open.

SABRINA—A CASE STUDY

Sabrina was a lovely little girl. She was bright and had a bubbly personality. But although she was only eight years old and had perfect vision, she was worried that she would some day have to wear glasses—and she didn't want to! In fact, Sabrina strongly stated that she never wanted to have glasses on her face. I discussed the little girl's concerns with her parents, and told them about the importance of drinking clean water, eating clean food, sunning the eyes, and exercising the eyes. (See the inset on page 64 of Chapter 4 for eye exercises.) Sabrina started her new eye-care routine and used it consistently as she matured. When the young girl graduated from high school, she sent me her high school graduation picture, and I did not see any glasses on her face. Coincidence? Maybe.

CONCLUSION

Remember, all things, even healthy things, can be overdone, but by using commonsense and utilizing the sun for your benefit, you can help your body detoxify, repair, and rebuild. Congratulations, you have completed step five on the road to awesome health.

Remember, Health is Wealth!

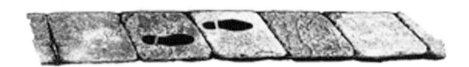

6. Posture

Avoiding the crooked road.

Posture is something that most of us give little thought to—until, for some reason, we succumb to back pain and wind up looking like a question mark. I saw many question marks come into my clinic throughout the years I was in practice, and I even saw patients crawling into my clinic on all fours due to some injury or, in too many cases, severe arthritis and osteoporosis. However, this is not the type of posture I'm talking about.

I am talking about everyday posture, which, if correct, will aid you in your quest to eliminate toxins and repair and rebuild your body. The acute postures I mentioned above required immediate treatment to get the patient out of pain and upright as soon as possible. Following this, I shared with the patient what I am now going to share with you—recommendations that will help optimize your health and prevent you from looking like a question mark in the future.

RHYTHMIC WALKING POSTURE

Let's first discuss the posture that will help you perform the rhythmic walking exercise discussed in Chapter 4. Keep your head up, eyes looking straight ahead, arms naturally swinging back and forth, and shoulders back, and use heel-to-toe walking at a quick but comfortable pace at which you can carry on a conversation. (No, this is not the military.) When you use good posture as you walk, you assist your body in receiving as much oxygen as possible by naturally expanding your rib cage. This allows more oxygen to saturate your bloodstream, which transports it to all the tissues of the body. And you know how important fresh oxygen is to your body.

STANDING POSTURE

Good standing posture is also vital to getting all the oxygen you need because it helps you avoid shallow breathing. (The average shallow breather takes in only a *fraction* of the air a deep breather receives.) What is the correct standing pos-ture? Stand straight and tall, eyes level with the horizon, palms facing your sides (not towards the rear), feet straight, and shoulders back. This will help keep your spine in line (okay, at ease) and, according to an old chiropractic saying, "When the spine is in line, you'll feel fine." This is worth remembering, since lack of alignment can cause the all-too-familiar misery of back pain. I have seen large men succumb to tears as a result of back pain. Keep your spine in line, and you'll avoid many tears.

SITTING POSTURE

It is also important to use good posture when sitting. Sit up straight with both feet on the floor, or, if more comfortable, rest your feet on a small box or step stool in front of you. I have found that placing a small pillow behind your lower back, between you and the chair, is an excellent way to maintain your posture while sitting or driving. Try to get out of the habit of crossing your legs while sitting. This habit not only will stress your spine by shifting the natural stress load placed upon it, but also diminish circulation to the legs. Many unfavorable looking veins and broken capillaries can be attributed to leg crossing.

For a moment, I would like to address men only. Many men carry wallets in their back pockets. (I carry a small one in my front pocket.) For this reason, they tend to sit upon a several-inch-thick piece of leather that is located under one side of their posterior. Consequently, they lean to one side when they sit. Even if the tilt is not noticeable to the eyes, the stress to the spine is very real because the spine has to compensate for the shift of weight caused by the wal-let. This added stress not only is unhealthy for your spine and surrounding musculature, but, by preventing your rib cage from fully expanding, impairs the amount of oxygen that enters your lungs. Like so many other bad postural habits, this keeps you from enjoying the full benefits of a normal oxygen sup-ply. Keep your wallet in a front pocket, and you'll remove this all-too-common obstacle to good health.

Now, talking to both men and women once again, let me suggest that if you are driving for a long distance, you get out of the car and walk around every couple of hours. If possible, stop at a rest area so that you can really stretch your legs. This will help restore proper blood flow throughout your legs and the rest of your body. Taking a deep breath of fresh air and getting more oxygen into your body is a wonderful way to instantly make yourself feel more alert and alive. I am not a big proponent of trying to set speed records on the way to Grandma's house. Give your body a break and take your time.

LIFTING OBJECTS

I am sure you have been told many times to "lift with your legs." This is good advice because the leg muscles are much stronger than the back muscles. The purpose of your leg muscles is to propel you forward when walking or running, to help lift the body upwards during climbing, and to assist your arms and back when lifting an object. The spinal muscles, on the other hand, are intended to provide support for the important spinal vertebrae, which house the even more important spinal cord. The spinal cord, which travels all the way up the spine and attaches to the brain, conducts sensory information from the peripheral nervous system to the brain, and from the brain to other parts of the body. Needless to say, the spinal cord is pretty important, so the bones and muscles that protect are important, too. Therefore, when you lift an object off the floor—even an object that is not very heavy—you must get into the habit of protecting your spine by squatting down with your legs, grasping the object, bringing it close to your stomach or chest, and then standing up. This simple habit will save your back from becoming injured. If the object is fairly heavy, I suggest getting help from someone trustworthy who can grab the other end of the object. Then squat down at the same time, move closer to the object, and stand up in unison.

One rule of thumb I used to tell my patients is that—regardless of the size, shape, or height of the object—it is vital to stand in front of the object when grasping it and then turn the feet and legs in the direction in which you want to move. Turn by moving your legs and feet—not by twisting your spine. So many people reach out and grab something with their body halfway turned towards where they want to go, and then twist themselves further as they grip the object. This motion puts a great deal of torque upon the lower back, and the lower back is not designed to twist.

Luggage Carrying Tip

When I walk through an airport, if I just have one bag to carry, I frequently use both arms to hold it up near my chest while walking. This allows me to cover greater distances without straining my back or arms. I have seen many people drag their suitcases behind them only to have someone else accidentally kick or stumble on the hand-pulled luggage, causing injuries to both parties. Plus, when pulling this type of luggage, you are causing a continual turning of the spine. Tell me that doesn't put stress on the muscles and joints of the back.

SPINAL BIOMECHANICS 101

Our entire spine has facet joints (also called apophyseal joints) that lock each spinal vertebra into those on either side. These facet joints interlock at approximately a 90-degree angle with one another in the lower back, a 60-degree angle in the middle back, and a 45-degree angle in the neck. Because of the angles of the facet joints, the lower back was designed to bend forward at the waist, bend slightly backward at the waist, and bend from side to side. It was not designed to rotate from side to side. According to an article presented in *The Journal of Bone and Joint Surgery*, "Joints which transmit a high proportion of intervertebral compression load through their apophyseal joints and which also have assymetrical facets, must be at great risk of developing degenerative changes and causing low back ache."[1] In short, this means that poor posture can and probably will cause arthritis.

AVOIDING DANGEROUS TWISTS AND TURNS

You now know that twisting the spine is a common way to cause back problems. Unfortunately, all too many things in life seem intent upon causing our backs to make unhealthy motions.

If you watch television, you've probably seen exercise commercials that promise a tighter tummy through use of a contraption that causes you to rotate your back from left to right. Switch channels, and you'll see an exercise gizmo that hyperextends the lower back. The problem with so many of these "tummy toners" is that twisting and hyperextending movements place a lot of stress on the lower back. I have seen many patients who hurt their spines using a "magic machine" to melt inches off their tummies. The truth is that it's really hard to beat floor exercises, which, when executed as explained in Chapter 4, tighten the stomach muscles effectively and safely.

Another threat to the back comes to us courtesy of Old Man Winter. When shoveling snow, many people bend over, grab a shovelful of snow, and throw the snow off to the side by moving the body upwards and sideways in a twisting motion. This is a surefire way to injure yourself. I always instructed my patients to slightly squat down with their legs and then push the snow with the shovel, or to throw a small amount of snow out in front of them onto the bank of snow, using their middle back to guide the throwing motion. As I mentioned earlier, whenever you move objects, you want to keep the objects in front of you and turn your lower body, not your spine. When shoveling snow, be sure to keep both your feet and your legs headed in the direction in which you want to throw the snow.

MATTRESSES

Many people wake up in the morning feeling more tired than they did when they went to bed. This demonstrates just how important a good night's rest is. And a vital component of a good night's rest is a good mattress.

Mattresses can be as individual as the person sleeping on them. Unfortunately, it is difficult to lie on a mattress in a department store for a few minutes and then decide which one is best for you. I've tried that. It's even harder to take a nap when there is so much hustle and bustle in the store. Fortunately, many mattress stores allow you to try out their products for a thirty- to ninety-day trial period in the comfort of your own home. Many will even deliver and set up the entire bed for you—including the frame and box spring—if you are interested in more than just a mattress. I generally recommended that my patients check out the mattresses that conform to the body, rather than the mattresses that force the body to conform to them.

Air mattresses allow you, at the touch of a button, to control how much or little support you receive on your side of the bed. I know of many couples who prefer this type of mattress as it allows one of the partners to have firmer support while the other one sleeps on a softer surface.

Water mattresses have come a long way since the big bladder effect of years ago. Once you were lying on those old-style water mattresses, it was quite a challenge to get out of bed, as you would sink below the bed frame. Today, a water mattress is composed of individual tubes that allow you to add or remove as much water as you like on each side of the bed. A good bit of effort is still required until you find the right comfort level, as the tubes are cumbersome to work with, and it generally takes two people to get the tubes filled with just the right amount of water to please the sleeper. But once the proper level of water has been found, it can be a very nice bed. The only regular maintenance required is placing an antifungal tablet in each tube once a year to inhibit fungal growth. I have personally slept on one of these mattresses for years.

Memory foam mattresses are also popular today. The foam is firm and conforms to the shape of your body, rather than forcing your body to conform to the bed. Also, there is very little movement on one sleeper's side of the bed when the other partner moves around. Assuming that you share your bed with someone else, this is an important consideration. The mattresses just discussed have baffle-type components which prevent the surface from bouncing as the result of someone else's movement. They also provide good support, so they are a great option for single sleepers as well as couples. (To learn more about getting a restful night's sleep, see Chapter 7.)

Journal Report

A study printed in the *Journal of Chiropractic Medicine* found that, "New bedding systems increased sleep quality and reduced back discomfort, factors that may be related to abatement of stress-related symptoms."[2] I think we can all appreciate how a quality mattress can make us feel in the morning. So if your back starts signaling that it's time to get a new mattress, listen to it.

SLEEPING POSTURES AND PILLOWS

Regardless of the type of mattress you use, you want to maintain good posture while sleeping. Most people favor one particular position when they rest, but unfortunately, some of these postures contribute to a poor night's rest, along with aches and pains in the morning.

If you are a back sleeper, one way to maintain good posture is to place a small pillow under your knees. This will take a great deal of pressure off your lower back and will result in a noticeable reduction of lower back discomfort in the morning.

If you sleep on your side, place a small pillow between your knees and another pillow between your arms. These pillows will greatly aid in maintaining spinal alignment. I have personally used pillows for years and have found them to be invaluable for a good night's sleep. Pillows can do wonders in compensating for a poor mattress, turn an average supportive mattress into a good mattress, and make a good mattress even better. Try using pillows before rushing out to get a new mattress. If the pillows don't relieve your morning back discomfort, look into one of the mattresses discussed earlier in the chapter.

Many patients told me that they moved around a lot when they slept. I would ask them how they knew they were moving around. After all, they were asleep. I never did get an answer to that one. Most people do change their position during the night, and many people wake at least once. If you find yourself waking up, I suggest that you readjust your pillows for greater comfort. A couple of hours of using pillows, even if the pillows wind up on the floor by morning, will make a big difference in how you feel upon awakening, and a well-rested body will definitely be better able to repair and rebuild itself.

Both back and side sleepers should use a pillow under their head. Don't laugh. Although this may sound obvious, I do know of people who don't place pillows under their head. The purpose of the pillow is to keep the head in line with the spine. Therefore, if you sleep on your back, your head should not be tilted so far forward that you can see your toes, nor should your head be tilted so far back that you can see the headboard of the bed. The head should be in a neutral position—aligned with the body. For side sleepers, the same spinal posture is suggested. You do not want your head to be tilted too far up or down on one side. You may want to ask someone to stand behind you while you are lying on your side to observe your posture. The observer should be able to mentally draw a straight line from the middle of the base of your skull to the base of your spine.

Generally, you don't need a thick pillow to keep your head aligned with your spine. I have found that most people use pillows that are too thick. When I check into a hotel for a conference, one of the first things I do—besides throwing the comforter on the floor because it is not very clean (how often do you wash your comforter?)—is remove the pillow from the pillowcase and replace it with a couple of thin bath towels. For me, there are few things as uncomfortable as trying to sleep with one of those overly high pillows wedged under my head.

If you are pregnant, I do not recommend sleeping on your back simply because this will cause the baby to place a great deal of pressure upon your arteries, veins, and blood vessels as he presses against the spine. This can make your blood vessels constrict and lead to high blood pressure. During pregnancy, it is far better to use a side-sleeping position.

And So It Was Said . . .

"I still need more healthy rest in order to work at my best. My health is the main capital I have and I want to administer it intelligently."
—ERNEST HEMINGWAY, NOVELIST

The one sleeping posture that I do not recommend is tummy sleeping. When you sleep on your stomach, your head is turned to one side, which puts a great deal of stress on the neck and upper back region of the spine, along with hyperextending your lower back. Earlier in the chapter, I mentioned that the neck was designed to rotate, but it was not meant to stay in one rotated position for several hours during sleep. I have treated many people who slept with their necks in a rotated position. Those patients were in a great deal of pain when they awoke because their neck muscles had locked up, and they could not turn their heads back to the center. They sure had a tough time driving to my clinic because not every route required just right-hand turns.

One of the reasons some people like to sleep on their stomachs is that they like the warmth of something pressing against the body. It's natural to want this, which is why I suggest sleeping on your side with a pillow not only between

Whiplash

Whiplash is an injury to the neck caused by rapid acceleration followed by rapid deceleration, such as that which occurs during an automobile accident. It is not only a spinal injury, but a soft tissue injury as well. Why am I discussing whiplash in a chapter on posture? Well, along with giving whiplash victims the treatment needed to restore neck curvature and thus alleviate the spinal and soft tissue symptoms, I would often send a patient home with an orthopedic neck pillow—a specially shaped pillow designed to help the patient create proper neck curvature by placing the neck in a slightly extended position during sleep. I would suggest that my patients try to sleep on their backs as much as possible rather than in a side posture, as this would help restore the proper curve.

The old saying, "If it ain't broke don't fix it!" doesn't always apply to healthcare, as prevention is important, but I do feel that it is not wise to use orthopedic pillows unless there is an existing problem. For that reason, once a patient's neck problem had been corrected, I always tried to wean him off the special neck pillow and replace it with the thinner pillow I recommend for regular use.

your knees, but also between your arms. The between-the-arms pillow provides warm pressure on the chest and tummy and creates proper spinal alignment. If you are a back sleeper and you want this warm pressure, I suggest placing and holding a pillow on top of your chest and stomach while sleeping. I have found, though, that back sleepers generally don't desire this type of pressure.

JIM—A CASE STUDY

Jim was a very active man both in his work and in his play. He was an electrician by day and liked to play tennis at night. He came to my clinic complaining of low back pain, which occurred mostly when he got up in the morning. As the day progressed, he seemed to feel quite well. I examined Jim and told him that there was nothing structurally wrong with his back. He simply needed to use a pillow at night when he slept. Jim was expecting to hear some big fancy diagnosis that he could tell his buddies back on the job site, but my recommendation was to place a pillow under or between his knees when he slept. Well, Jim took my advice and the back pain that he experienced in the morning subsided. I don't know what he told his buddies.

CHARLES—A CASE STUDY

Charles came to my clinic at the urging of his family. His health was deteriorating. He had gained quite a bit of weight over the years, and his ankles had swelled through fluid retention. His joints ached, his skin had lost much of its color, and he had problems sleeping because of sleep apnea. He was also tired all the time. His wife and family said that they wanted Charles to be with them for a long time to come. His daughter was especially sad because she was planning on getting married within the year and was afraid that Dad would not be there.

After examining Charles and looking at all those checked boxes on his patient form, I treated his aches and pains, which made him feel a bit more comfortable. I then told his family that if he followed my advice, he would not only be able to attend his daughter's wedding, but also enjoy the first dance with her at the reception. I explained that Charles would need to implement some simple lifestyle changes. Clean water and organic, natural food, gentle rhythmic and strengthening exercises, twenty-four-hour weekly fasts, twenty-minute daily sunnings, and good posture while sleeping would make a world of difference.

I outlined Charles' program, and monitored him once a week for two months, and once a month after that. By month six, he was becoming a changed man. One year later, the old Charles was back and better than ever. He walked his daughter down the aisle, and he did get that first dance in. The problem now wasn't the first dance—it was how to get Dad off the dance floor because he was having so much fun.

SLEEP APNEA

I would like to address sleep apnea, a condition in which breathing halts briefly during sleep, causing the individual to wake up. I have found that sleep apnea is commonly a result of sinus problems, asthma issues, excess weight, and/or a weakening of the stomach and throat muscles. It is my experience, too, that sleep apnea is more common with people who sleep on their back rather than their side.

If you suffer from sleep apnea, try following the advice presented in the earlier chapters of this book. By improving your diet; walking, which results in weight loss; doing curl-ups, which strengthens stomach and throat muscles; and drinking clean water, which helps your body detoxify, you can help make your sleep apnea a thing of the past. Until the problem is corrected, I suggest sleeping on your side.

FEET AND POSTURE

There are too many people with foot problems, which in turn, affect their posture. Something as simple as walking barefoot can help strengthen your feet and prevent you from getting the many foot maladies that are so common today. The journal *Arthritis & Rheumatism* published an article that suggested, "Modern shoes and walking practices may need to be reevaluated with regard to their effects on the prevalence and progression of osteoarthritis in our society."[3] This is just what I am going to be talking about next.

We have been told for years to keep our shoes on because we'll hurt our feet if we go barefoot. Let's not forget, however, that before the invention of shoes, people walked miles upon bare feet. Even once shoes were invented, some people could not afford them. It was thousands of years before even cheap sandals were worn.

When you walk barefoot, you strengthen, not weaken, the muscles of your feet. The strengthening prevents your arches from "falling" (flat feet) and also helps prevent an assortment of other foot maladies, such as pronation (excessive inward rolling of the ankle), supination (excessive outward rolling of the ankle), bunions (an arthritic bump on the side of the big toe), ligament sprains, and foot muscle and tendon strains.

When walking barefoot, stay on surfaces that are clear of potentially damaging debris. Dirt trails, the beach, the lawn, or the garden are preferable to streets and sidewalks. In Chapter 5, I talked about the importance of the sun. One reason the sun is so important for your well-being is that it emits a lot of healthful electromagnetic energy, which can be used by the body. The Earth also emits this energy, so by walking barefoot on a lawn or beach you soak up the Earth's natural electromagnetic frequency. What a wonderful combination of sun and Earth power.

I realize that it just isn't practical to go barefoot all day, but I see no reason why most of us can't go barefoot or at least in stocking feet at home. Strong feet will help keep your spine in line, affecting your posture in a very positive way, and will ultimately allow you to get more of that precious oxygen that will help detoxify, repair, and rebuild your body. (To learn more about going barefoot, see page 159 in Chapter 15.)

INVERSION

One great way to improve your posture and give your spine a break from the pressure caused by standing, sitting, and walking is to invert yourself—turn yourself upside down—for five to fifteen minutes a day. I suggested this to my patients who wanted to maintain good posture, and especially to those who suf-

Staying Tall

Inversion therapy is great if you are concerned about losing height. As we get older, our discs lose some of their fluid due to aging and gravity. We all experience it. The compression of discs is accelerated by the onset of osteoporosis and osteoarthritis. This results in people getting slightly shorter. Inversion therapy helps relieve the downward pressure on the discs, slowing the loss of fluid.

fered from some postural/spinal problem. Many of my patients incorporated some type of inversion therapy into their health program and reported that their spinal problems were greatly alleviated.

Inversion, or "upside down" therapy, has been around for years. An individual lies on a padded board hooking his ankles under a bar, and gently tips the board backwards. He can then simply invert himself to a near vertical position with his head pointing toward the floor. Inversion is a great way to take pressure off the spinal nerves and especially the discs, which act as shock absorbers between the vertebrae. It is also a great way to aid the flow of spinal fluid, which carries nutrients to the brain and spinal cord. When you are inverted for a few minutes and return to an upright position, your spine feels wonderfully relaxed and free of tension, and your posture naturally improves. I stand just a bit taller after having been on an inversion board.

I own a slant cushion, which is an inexpensive cushion that slants at a 45-degree angle, much like a big wedge. I lay with my head at the bottom of the cushion and my feet at the top, and it feels wonderful, although I am not completely inverted. However you achieve an inversion, and whether it is partial or complete, the point is to relax and relieve built-up pressure on the spine. Inversion and body-slant therapy work! I have heard of people actually increasing their height by being inverted on a consistent daily basis. No, it won't make you six feet tall if you now top out at five feet five inches, but an increase of up to an inch in height over time is not all that uncommon.

BABIES AND POSTURE

Now let's move on and discuss one of my favorite topics: Babies. I just love babies! I saw many babies in my years of practice. When parents brought a newborn to me, I would advise them to have the infant sleep on his side with a foam support both in front of his spine and behind it to keep him from rolling over. When a baby sleeps on his side and he spits up during sleep, the contents rolls

GLADYS—A CASE STUDY

Gladys was a wiry little lady at the young age of eighty-five. She came to my clinic stating that she was having middle back pain. Over the years, Gladys had developed a small hump on her mid-back. A real get-to-the-point kind of gal, she indicated the hump and said, "Doc, that's where it hurts!" I said it was nice to meet her as I stuck out my hand to shake hers. Then she said, "What are you going to do about it!?" As I said, there was no time for cordial hellos. I explained that she was experiencing arthritis and osteoporosis in her spine, and that she needed to start eating and drinking clean foods and water along with getting some sunlight. I also suggested that she begin a program of inversion therapy. She said, "Doctor Senne, how can hanging by my ankles help the pain in my back?" I convinced her to try the slant cushion—no hanging by the ankles necessary, I assured her.

I treated Gladys and as she left my clinic, she shook my hand and said she would follow my suggestions and give that upside-down thing a try. Gladys returned to my clinic one week later. She was now six feet four . . . just kidding. I walked into the treatment room and once again I didn't get a handshake, I got a hug! She told me her back pain was gone! She still had her hump, though, and not one to mince words, she said, "Dr. Senne, what are you going to do about my hump?" I told her that the hump took a long time to get there and might take some time to correct itself. To this day, she faithfully inverts herself, and her hump has diminished.

out onto the crib as opposed to running back into the little one's throat, which can happen if the child is lying on his back. I do not recommend that children sleep on their stomachs because an infant can press his tiny nose and mouth right into the mattress, resulting in suffocation. I have found that the foam supports work quite well in keeping infants in place during sleep.

Many parents would ask me if they should place a pillow under their child's head, and I always recommended that they skip the pillow until the child was old enough to be out of the crib. A pillow can easily cause a little one to suffocate. If you're wondering why the foam support doesn't pose a suffocation risk, there are two reasons. First, the Velcro at the bottom of the support secures it to the bedding, which keeps both the support and the child from moving around. Second, these supports are fairly firm, so they can't really get pressed closely against an infant's face, shutting air out.

I also do not encourage parents to place blankets or other soft objects in the crib, as they also can lead to suffocation. Simply dress your child as warmly as needed. If you opt to use a bumper around the inside of the crib, make sure it is fastened tightly and checked daily for any loosened strings. Also make sure that the sheet is tucked in very tightly to prevent any sheet pockets from forming in the crib. As we all know, as infants get older and stronger, they move around a lot during sleep. At that point, the foam supports will no longer keep them in place and can be removed from the crib. The infant will often go into a tummy-sleeping posture, which is okay because his neck flexibility will permit him to handle neck rotation for an extended period of time. Babies seek warm pressure upon their little bodies, which is why it is so important to keep the crib as clutter free as possible. Once the baby is past the spit-up stage—usually when he begins to sleep through the night—back sleeping is fine.

INFANT DEVELOPMENT

When working with parents and their babies, I always told parents that they should not encourage their kids to walk before they were ready. I know that sounds odd. Many excited parents rush out to buy these tiny walkers for their baby so they can stand up all the time and oh, those cute little baby shoes! I believe that each baby should have the freedom to stand and walk when he is ready. It is good—and actually very necessary—for babies to crawl. There is a reason that babies develop the way they do, and sometimes the less we interfere with this developmental process, the better it is for the child.

When a baby crawls, he is developing the proper spinal curvature for his body, and also developing his brain. The right side of the brain controls the left side of the body and vice versa, so as a child uses his right leg, his right arm, etc., he matures the opposite side of the brain. When you force or encourage a baby to be upright within his first few months of life, you don't allow his spinal curvature to develop properly, and you don't promote proper brain development. Very early walking also places too much stress on tiny feet and legs. Generally speaking, the longer a baby crawls, the fewer back, leg, and joint problems he will develop over his lifetime. I have seen the proud look on parents' faces when they show people how quickly Junior was able to stand. Parents that work with their little one daily so that he will be the first on the block to stand on his own often find that Junior suffers from bowed legs, collapsed arches, or other leg and foot problems as he grows. Now, I am not saying that you shouldn't assist your child as he learns to walk. I am simply saying that although those upright baby scooters are fun, your child shouldn't be kept in them all day. Allow your child to crawl until *he* decides that it's time to stand and walk.

Before your baby walks, keep him barefoot as much as possible. I realize that out in public, you may at times want to place shoes on your baby—although socks are better—but at home, let your baby go barefoot. Once your baby has naturally progressed to standing on his own, encourage him to walk barefoot, as well. Barefoot walking will make those little baby feet become strong and supportive. If you can help develop strength in your baby's little foot muscles, his feet will be able to support his body, and he will experience better posture and fewer foot, leg, and back problems as he grows older.

CONCLUSION

As a healthcare practitioner, one of my main objectives was to get my patients' bodies back in tune with Nature. I utilized therapies that aided their bodies in becoming "recharged' with Nature's natural energy, which emanates from the sun and Earth. I used to have fun with my patients and tell them it was time for them to get their batteries charged up. They definitely understood about their body's natural frequency, the Earth's and sun's frequencies, and how our Creator designed everything to work together.

If you follow the recommendations outlined in this book, you will have far fewer aches and pains in your spine and your corresponding joints, and you will help your body avoid spinal and joint problems in the future. Good posture will also enable you to benefit from more life-giving, cleansing oxygen. In other words, you will be well on your way to attaining and maintaining your health. You have just completed step six on the road to long-lasting health.

Remember, Health is Wealth!

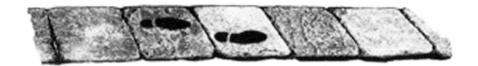

7. Sleeping and Resting

Flowing with the rhythm of life.

I used to keep pushing my body, no matter how tired I felt. "I'm young," I thought. "I can handle it." But my body finally rebelled and, despite a waiting room full of patients, I was forced to rest.

You know how wonderful it feels to awaken from a good night's sleep. Your body, mind, soul, and even social and emotional well-being are recharged and ready to take on the challenges of a new day. Ever wonder why it is generally more difficult to fall asleep and feel rested when you are forced to sleep during the day rather than the night? This occurs because the human body functions most efficiently when it is allowed to conform to the rhythms of life and to follow a similar routine on a daily basis. Going to bed at about the same time each night, waking up at the same time each morning, eating at the same time each day, and exercising at the same time each day all help the body function at its best. This chapter will further explain daily rhythms and give you some tips for getting the rest and relaxation that your body requires.

THE RHYTHM OF LIFE

The human body follows its own circadian rhythm—a twenty-four-hour cycle of activity that is optimal for overall health. When this rhythm gets interrupted because you ignore or are unable to follow it, the detoxification, repairing, and rebuilding of the body is severely hampered. You may know people who work night shifts or some type of inconsistent work hours—two weeks of working days followed by two weeks of working nights, for instance. These odd hours disrupt eating and sleeping patterns, resulting in health problems. According to an article in *The American Journal of Psychiatry*, "Changes in an individual's routines that are apparently benign from a psychological stress standpoint can place considerable stress on the body's attempt to maintain synchronized sleep/wake, appetite, energy, and alertness rhythms."[1] I have found this to be very true.

The rhythm of life coincides not only with a twenty-four-hour timespan, but also with a monthly timespan. In my clinic, I used to see women who were experiencing menstrual irregularities and were frustrated because they wanted to start a family. I noticed that many of these women worked night shifts or some other irregular shift. When these women changed back to regular day shifts for an extended period of time, their monthly cycle tended to become more regular, and their fertility improved. According to an article in *Applied Ergonomics,* "Shift work, in particular night work, can have a negative impact on health and well-being as it can cause disturbances of the normal circadian rhythyms . . . beginning with the sleep/wake cycle. . . . Shift and night work may have more specific adverse effects on women's health in relation to their particular hormonal and reproductive function."[2]

I suggest that as far as possible, any woman with menstruation problems get on a regular schedule that conforms to the circadian rhythms of working during the day and sleeping at night. Along with using coconut oil rubs, eating seed-containing produce, and consuming other clean foods, this can help establish regular menstruation and fertility.

A BABY'S RHYTHM OF LIFE

Natural life rhythms should be supported as soon as a baby is born. All children, babies included, seem to thrive on a consistent schedule. I am not a big proponent of feeding a baby whenever she wants to be fed, letting her sleep whenever she desires to sleep, and playing whenever she wants to play. This can result in fussy babies who exhaust both their parents and themselves. I know many parents who let their little one eat and sleep whenever she wants, and then wonder why she is so cranky and difficult. Very likely, it is due to the lack of a healthy schedule.

If you can establish a routine right away with your baby, your whole family will be happier. Feed your child at approximately the same times each day, follow this with a period of wakefulness, and then place the baby in her crib so that she can sleep—again, at a consistent time. Your baby will then know what to expect and when to expect it.

You can develop a routine with your child very early in life. For example, my wife breast-fed our daughter at regular times, and later on gave solid foods to her at about the same times each day. Our daughter would want to sleep while eating, as many babies do, but my wife would tickle her to keep her awake. For the first two months of her life, my daughter was fed on a three-hour cycle. During the day, the first part of the three hours was feeding time, followed by about one hour of awake time. The remainder of the three hours was sleep time. During the night, we woke her every three hours for a feeding and put her right back in the crib, with no play time between eating and sleeping. After eight weeks, we no longer awakened our daughter every three hours for a feeding, and she got six to seven hours of uninterrupted sleep during the night. By thirteen weeks, she was sleeping nine to ten hours a night.

After about the sixteenth month, many babies drop one of their daytime naps, but that doesn't mean that the child shouldn't be kept on a regular schedule. It simply means that the periods of wakefulness becomes longer.

WHAT IS A GOOD NIGHT'S SLEEP?

Newborn infants need the greatest amount of sleep—about twelve to sixteen hours a day, including naps. As discussed above, after the first sixteen months or so, little ones require slightly less sleep.

After infancy, children are still growing and need at least ten hours of sleep per night, and even more if possible. After the onset of puberty, kids should get at least nine hours of sleep per night. Once people reach their early to mid-twenties, about six to nine hours of sleep is optimal. (I happen to lean towards eight hours.) Your daily pursuits—including mental, physical, spiritual, social, and emotional activities—will help determine the amount of sleep that you require.

The Importance of REM

Every night, the body goes through five stages of sleep. One of these stages is called REM, or rapid eye movement sleep. This form of sleep is important to your body because it allows you to dream. Most adults who have a healthy night of rest spend about 20 percent of it in REM sleep. (Children spend more time in the REM stage.) Those who don't get a good night's sleep and, therefore, experience little or no REM cycle, suffer from a host of physical, mental, social, and emotional problems. Beginning on page 100, this chapter will guide you in getting a beneficial night of rest that includes all the stages of sleep.

In this busy world, most of us use an alarm clock to wake up, rather than relying on a natural "alarm." Our Creator intended us to awaken when the sun comes up and sleep when the sun goes down, but in a world of artificial lights and modern comforts, humans have altered their rest patterns. I am a big proponent of the old saying, "Early to bed and early to rise." I can't adequately emphasize the importance of performing most of your activities during daylight hours and at around the same time each day. The more you follow this schedule, the more likely it is that your body will adjust and gently nudge you when it's time to rest, eat, exercise, and work. You'll be amazed by how accurately your body will guide you from activity to activity. In fact, you often won't need a watch because your body will instinctively know what time it is. For many years, I did not even own a wristwatch. I have one now, but seldom wear it. Maybe that is why I am always late for my own lectures! Just kidding, but many people have commented on the fact that, despite my very busy life, I do not rely on a watch. I guess my body is attuned to the rhythms of my life.

HOW CAN YOU GET A GOOD NIGHT'S SLEEP?

Despite the body's need for rest, many people have trouble sleeping. When people don't take care of themselves, eat nutrient-poor foods, ignore the need to detoxify through fasting, enjoy little to no exercise, get inadequate amounts of sunshine, have poor posture, and lack fresh air and clean water, it is no wonder that sleeping becomes difficult. Many people now need a pill to go to sleep, and some need a pill to wake up, as well. Some keep taking pills during the day to calm them down, pep them up, or improve performance. This isn't a life I would want to have. But as already discussed, adequate sleep is important. An article in the *Journal of Clinical Sleep Medicine* stated, "Sleep loss may be differentially disruptive to regions of the brain."[3] Fortunately, as the remainder of this discussion will show, there are healthier steps you can take to get a good night's sleep.

Enjoy a Healthy Lifestyle

The best way to get the sleep you need *without* the aid of sleeping pills is to follow the lifestyle recommendations presented earlier in the book and then establish a consistent daily routine. Healthy food, clean water, weekly fasting, sunshine, good posture, and the other lifestyle components already discussed will help prevent the physical problems that can keep you from sleeping. An exercise program will help you fall asleep and will even improve the quality of your rest. And, of course, a regular schedule of activities will let your body know when it's time to go to bed.

Don't Eat Right Before Bed

Try not to get into the habit of eating food right before you go to sleep. You will want your body to rest without having to digest your latest snack or meal. A good night's rest is, in some manner, like a mini-fast because it gives your body time to detoxify, repair, and rebuild. (Just remember that a good night's sleep is no substitute for a twenty-four-hour fast, as discussed in Chapter 3.) If you should wake up during the night, feel free to grab a glass of water with a dash of lemon, as this will further aid detoxification without burdening your body with food.

Clear Your Mind for Sleep

Many people mentally review their day while in bed. It's true that no matter how busy you get with the demands of work, family, and friends, you need time alone for a short period each day to plan, evaluate, and think about your day, your week, your month, your year—and yes, your life. I like to say, "Failing to plan is planning to fail." Just keep in mind that it is far better to review your day and clear your thoughts *before* getting into bed. Then, when you get into bed, you will be ready for sleep.

I personally have found that as I review my day, it is a wonderful opportunity to call upon my Creator, give thanks for my many blessings, and pray for strength of body, guidance of mind, calmness of emotions, friendships for my social well-being, and peace within my soul. This is a personal choice, but I am amazed by the feeling I get when I call upon someone greater than myself.

Darken and Quiet the Room

When you retire at night, I suggest that you darken the room. This will help your body fall sleep. If you awaken during the night, do not turn on the brightest lights in the house. When you close your eyes to sleep, the pineal gland in the center of the brain starts to release a hormone called melatonin. This hormone actually aids you in falling asleep by making you drowsy. During the night, the output of melatonin is progressively lessened so that you will wake up as morning approaches. If you turn on bright lights during the night, your melatonin production will be interrupted, making it more difficult for you to fall back asleep. So make your bedroom dark and keep it dark, using just a small night-light in a hallway to illuminate your path.

It is also important to make your bedroom as quiet as possible, unplugging the phone and closing the door if necessary. Some people prefer a fan or some type of "white noise" in the room, but I feel that the quieter the room is, the more rest your mind will receive because it will not have to work to block out sound.

Enjoy Clean Air

Slightly open a window in your bedroom so that you get fresh air as you sleep. Many of us work in a climate-controlled building all day. When you breathe in fresh air at night, it will be delivered to your cells where it is need-ed for detoxifying, repairing, and rebuilding. I actually recommend keeping the window cracked open *all the time* so that you continually allow fresh air to enter your home. This will not adversely affect your heating and cooling bills. If you live in a smog-filled city, purchase an inexpensive window ventilator that will fit right under your open window and filter the air as it flows into your home. This will help keep your environment free of dust, pollen, dirt, and smoke.

Be aware that fresh air is also great for your skin, acting as a sort of air bath. For this reason, when you sleep, you should wear loose-fitting clothing or nothing at all. When your skin is able to fully breathe, free from suffocating clothing, your body will be better able to detoxify through its pores.

SUSAN—A CASE STUDY

Susan was a new patient who arrived for her appointment at my clinic about an hour late. When she handed me her filled-out patient questionnaire, I saw that she had checked most of the boxes. She said she felt a little embarrassed by all the checks, but I told her to relax because that was the reason she had come to my clinic in the first place. If she felt great, she wouldn't be there.

I got to know Susan a little better when she told me about her work and rest patterns. Her days varied from one extreme to another. She was an executive for a big company and felt that she was never caught up with all her work. On some nights, she would go to bed at midnight. The next evening, exhausted, she would fall into bed at 8:00 PM. Some days, she ate breakfast at 7:00 AM; on other days, there was no time for breakfast. Lunch was eaten only when she could fit it in. Sometimes, she just snacked all day and grabbed a fast dinner.

One of the first ideas I shared with Susan was that she needed to create a healthy daily lifestyle routine. I told her that if she didn't start taking care of herself, eventually, she wouldn't be able to do her job at all no matter how committed she was to her career. Following my examination and treatment for her aches and pains, I discussed the steps she must take to create a healthier lifestyle.

Susan implemented the advice given earlier in this book regarding clean water and food, weekly twenty-four-hour fasts, daily walks in the sunshine, proper sleeping posture, eight hours of sleep a night, and, of course, a daily rhythm. A couple of months went by before I saw Susan at a conference that I was attending. I asked her to stop by my clinic just to fill out another symptom survey form so we could compare the checked boxes with those on the original sheet. A few days later, Susan arrived at my clinic on time. After she filled out the second form, we found that she had significantly fewer problems than she had been experiencing at the initial visit. Since then, Susan has continued on the road to health and has been very happy about her lifestyle changes.

Keep Electronic Devices Out of the Bedroom

When you sleep, try to keep electronic devices out of your bedroom, or at least as far from your head as possible. If you use a plug-in electric digital alarm clock, for instance, do not keep it on your bedside table, but place it far away from your body. Why? Studies have shown that specific negative EMF (electromagnetic field) radiation is emitted by devices such as electric alarm clocks, cell phones, television sets, microwaves, and computers. While it is nice to have these modern-day conveniences, they may not be all that healthy for you, because the EMF radiation can enter the body and disrupt its natural electromagnetic field. In fact, EMF waves are another source of toxins in your life, just like harmful chemicals. The old warning "Don't sit so close to the TV" was really good advice. Now, I don't think that you need to dispense with these conveniences, but it is good to keep as many as possible out of the bedroom—or at least at a good distance from you—so that your sleeping environment is as toxin-free as you can make it. (For more information on household electricity, see Chapter 17.)

MAGNETICS AND SLEEP

You have just read several tips for getting a good night's sleep. Here's another thought: If at all possible, place your bed so that your head is pointing north. Sounds silly doesn't it? As you know, the Earth has north and south poles. (I know what you're thinking . . . thanks for the geography lesson.) But human beings also have a magnetic field produced by the motion of electric charges. By aligning your body with the north while you sleep, you can actually enhance your own magnetic field and attain a radiant glow of health and vibrancy.

There are some bedrooms that can't accommodate a north-facing bed. In that case, I often recommend that people sleep on a magnetic mattress pad. This is a foam pad with magnets sewn into the foam. It creates the same effect as aligning yourself with the north pole.

When in practice, I routinely gave small magnets to my patients to take home with them. I would place the north side of one magnet on one side of the body part I was treating, and the south side of another magnet on the opposite side of that body part. This was something patients could also do for themselves once they saw how it should be done. Since the magnets were small, they worked well on knee, ankle, wrist, and elbow pain. Oftentimes, I wrapped magnets either under or over a cast or other type of wrap to promote healing of a broken bone, strained muscle, or sprained ligament or tendon. Magnets have a wonderful ability to decrease inflammation and speed the healing process by realigning the positive and negative ions (charges) of the respective cells.

Magnets Doing Their Magic

The Baylor College of Medicine tested the effects of magnets on healing. They concluded, "The majority of patients in the study who received treatment with a magnet, reported significant decrease in pain."[4] Now, magnets are not a cure-all, but they can certainly assist the body's healing process. Just be aware that standing closer to the magnets on your refrigerator door won't heal you.

I realize that some people will implement every piece of advice presented in this book, while others will pick and choose the suggestions they feel they can incorporate into their life. It is my hope that you will adopt as many recommendations as possible. Even if you follow only one suggestion, your health will benefit greatly, which will make you consider further lifestyle changes. One day, you may even sleep with your head pointing north.

ALLERGIES AND SLEEP

Many people experience congestion and other allergic symptoms in the morning, only to have these symptoms recede as the day progresses. They probably don't realize that the cause of this problem may be their bedding. The unpleasant fact is that many beds are home to microscopic "critters" called dust mites. Dust mites—which are too small to see without a microscope—feed on the flakes of shed human skin that accumulate in bedding, as well as in your favorite easy chair, couch, and carpets. If you don't wash your sheets, pillowcases, and blankets daily—and most people don't—the dust mites settle into this hospitable environment. And dust mite allergy is a major cause of congestion, sneezing, and other unpleasant symptoms in many people.

I like to sleep on organic cotton sheets and pillowcases, and use a special allergy-free mattress cover to help eliminate dust mites. Because wool is a great dust mite deterrent, I also use a wool pillow within my pillowcase. Mattresses that contain wool also help to keep dust mites away, although a wool mattress is more costly than an allergy-free mattress cover. I generally recommend that adults use allergy-free covers and that infants sleep on wool mattresses. A little wool crib mattress is much less expensive than a full-size mattress and ensures that no suffocation hazard could occur due to air pockets forming in the allergy-free cover. I also recommend that you wash your bedding at least once a week, if not more often. After all, do you wear the same clothes every day?

What about the dust mites that can live on your upholstered furniture? Simple, attractive, washable throws can be tossed over couches and chairs to help eliminate the dust mite problem. Just be sure to launder them frequently.

PETS AND SLEEP

Ah pets! We love our pets, and they can be wonderful companions. There are pets that stay inside the house much of the time, and others that primarily stay outside. If your pets stay outside most of the time but come in for the night, I suggest that you avoid letting them sleep on your bed. Pets have a tendency to carry pollen, mites, fleas, dander, and other allergens in their fur, especially if they are outside much of the time. (If you are allergic to dander, of course, that will be present even in indoor pets.) You may want to tell Fluffy that she should sleep in her own doggie bed. Or perhaps you can sleep on the couch whenever Flufyy insists on sleeping in your bed. Then wash the sheets the next day, after Fluffy has gone out to play.

To help avoid flea infestations—both in your bed and elsewhere in your house—place an all-natural herbal flea collar on your pet or massage some garlic oil into your pet's fur. Garlic is a wonderful deterrent to many of the pests that want to live in fur. It's important to avoid conventional flea collars because commonly used chemical repellents such as permethrin and diazinon can lead to toxic buildup in your pet. The United States Environmental Protection Agency has stated that it's vital to choose flea collars carefully "due to concerns over safety issues based on thousands of adverse effects incidents investigated by the EPA."[5]

Finally, although this is not directly related to the subject of sleeping, I feel it is important to recommend that you keep everything for your pets as natural and healthful as possible. If your cat uses a litter box, buy litter that is wheat-, alfalfa-, wood chip-, or newspaper-based—not clay-based litter, which contains the toxic chemical crystalline silica. Feed your pets clean, pure water, and natural or organic pet food from a bag versus a can (avoid aluminum). Make sure that they get in some exercise. Pets are important members of the family, and can profit from the same healthful lifestyle that will benefit you. Of course, getting Fluffy to sleep with her head facing north may be a bit of a challenge.

Organic Sheets

Did you know that many people are allergic to the fiber makeup of their bed sheets? Organic sheets, and in particular cotton sheets, are a great way to avoid the allergy problems that bed sheets so often cause. You spend about one third of your life sleeping, so doesn't it make sense to sleep in the most wholesome environment possible?

RESTING AND RELAXING

So far, this chapter has presented a wealth of tips for getting healthful nighttime sleep, but it's also important to get in some rest and relaxation during the day. I realize that you probably don't have the luxury of meditating in a meadow full of sunshine, flowers, and bunnies, but it is important to consider the benefits of fitting some relaxation into your busy schedule.

Many people move at such a frenetic pace all day that when they do fall into bed, their minds are traveling so fast that they simply can't turn off their thoughts. This is yet another reason why so many people toss and turn at night. On page 101, I talked about the need to clear your mind right before you go to sleep, but it's also helpful to unwind for a few minutes during the day. Many countries, such as Spain and Mexico, actually encourage businesses to close during the day so that employees can take an afternoon nap, or siesta. Now, I can't imagine most Americans closing their stores and offices so they can nap, but I do suggest taking a ten- to fifteen-minute break when you are not eating or drinking, so that you can sit down and perform a few deep breathing exercises. Better yet, go for a gentle stroll outside in the fresh air and sun, breathe deeply, and let your mind and body relax. This is a great way to do a short detoxification, repair, and rebuilding. You will feel recharged, will be more productive during the day, and yes, you will rest better at night.

CONCLUSION

Sleep is a great way to detoxify, repair, and rebuild your body for today, tomorrow, and the week ahead. Both nighttime sleep and daytime relaxation benefit your body, mind, emotions, social well-being, and soul. Happy resting! You have just completed step seven on the road to amazing health.

Remember, Heath is Wealth!

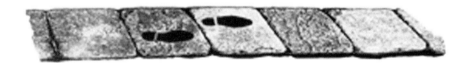

8. Bowel Health

Can we talk about something else?

The importance of regularly eliminating body waste cannot be underestimated. My symptom questionnaire asked patients how often they had bowel movements, and it was not uncommon for people to tell me that they hadn't had a bowel movement in three days, or even a week! For the most part, they were not upset by this state of affairs because they had been told that everyone had his own biological rhythm, and that Nature tells you when it's time to go. Unfortunately, that type of thinking can cause people to suffer needlessly with health disorders.

Of course, not everyone has such a casual attitude toward elimination. Many people take laxatives to help them go to the bathroom more often and also to help soften their stool. These unnatural stimulants force the body to excrete waste when it may not be ready to do so. That's why people often end up taking another pill or potion so that they can *stop* going to the bathroom. What a cycle! While I enjoy spending time in a warm, relaxing bath, I would not appreciate having to use the bathroom repeatedly for this reason. This is yet another situation in which people use man-made products to replace the work of Nature.

What is good bowel health and how can you establish and maintain it? This chapter will first discuss bowel basics and then guide you in making lifestyle choices that will help you keep your bowel—and your entire digestive system—in good working order for maximum health and well-being.

ELIMINATION 101

The process of digestion breaks down the solid and liquid foods you consume into simple substances (nutrients) that can be utilized by your body. Eventually, the bloodstream carries these nutrients from the digestive system to all the cells and organs, including the liver, which helps remove any remaining toxins from the blood. Any solid substances that cannot be used by the body are eventually moved into the large intestine (colon), where they are stored for a short period of time and then excreted as feces. Any liquid substances that are not needed by the body are filtered by the kidneys and moved into the bladder, where they are stored for a short period of time and then excreted as urine. These waste products (especially feces) are loaded with toxins, so the process of elimination removes not only unwanted materials, but also materials that can actually injure the body. Therefore, regular elimination is one of Nature's many ways of keeping you healthy.

Above, I mentioned that solid waste should remain in the colon for only a short period of time. What do I mean by "short"? People who have a bowel movement once a week or even every few days should certainly be more regular. Ideally, they should have a bowel movement about a half an hour to an hour after each meal. At these times, when the body is functioning properly, strong muscle contractions move down the length of the colon, pushing the waste forward and expelling it from the body.

When I discuss the frequency with which bowel movements should occur, people often exclaim, "Dr. Senne, I would spend my whole day in the bathroom!" Well, you don't have to be in there all day if you do your business and get out. If you make it a habit of going to the restroom within an hour after eating and you simply relax, something usually will happen. I also suggest that you place your feet on a small footstool that's only a few inches high during the elimination process. This position will allow you to better push down on your colon, and therefore assist you in moving your bowels.

One more bowel "basic" should be mentioned. When waste moves into the colon, it contains a good deal more water than it usually does when it's expelled as stool. In the colon, some of this water is removed from the waste, making the feces firmer. If the waste remains in the colon too long, the colon can remove too much water, resulting in feces that are hard, dry, and difficult to pass. When this situation persists, it is known as constipation.

Go When You Have to Go

You should not hold in a bowel movement unless you have no bathroom available. When you hold in your bowel movements, the body quits sending the colon signals to evacuate, and the colon keeps removing fluid from the stool, making it uncomfortably dry and potentially painful to pass.

CARLY—A CASE STUDY

Carly, a lady in her mid-thirties, visited my clinic because she was experiencing bouts of dizziness. She mentioned that she had been bothered by this symptom for about two months, and that the dizziness was increasing in frequency.

As I was examining Carly, I asked her how often she used the restroom to have a bowel movement. I took her a little off guard, and she looked at me with a surprised expression. I didn't mean to get personal, but I needed to get personal. She stated that she used the restroom faithfully, every three days. Now it was my turn to be surprised. Only every three days? No wonder she was experiencing dizziness. It was caused by a buildup of toxic wastes in her system.

Carly related that she was sometimes just too busy to use the restroom. She babysat several children during the day, and she felt that she needed to attend to their needs before attending to her own. I told her that while I admired her dedication to her job, it was important that when Nature called, she heeded the call! "If you don't get on a regular elimination schedule, you will one day be too sick too care for any children," I explained. I proceeded to treat her for a "stuck-open" ileocecal valve. (See page 111 for a discussion of this valve.) Carly used the restroom after this procedure and said she felt better. I advised her to perform the lymphatic massage every day to help keep her valve working properly. She did this, and her dizziness went away. She also listened to Nature more closely and made it a daily habit to use the restroom. Her dizziness did not return.

KEEPING YOUR BOWEL IN GOOD WORKING ORDER

You now know a little about how the bowel works, or at least how it should work. If your system is not acting as it should—or if you want to do all you can to keep your bowel in tiptop condition—your lifestyle should include several important components. One of these components is appropriate food, and the other is lymphatic massage.

Choosing Foods That Promote Bowel Health

Our Creator made us unique in many ways. Four-legged animals have colons that are pretty much straight tubes, allowing waste to move easily. Because we stand on two legs, we have a colon that is shaped much like an upside-down U with right-angled corners. This can make it a bit harder to pass waste along the length of the colon and down into the anus for expulsion. Fiber, which is indigestible, modifies the consistency of stool by adding bulk to it, making it easier to pass. Therefore, the more fruits and vegetables you eat, the better your bowel will work and the faster your waste will be eliminated. In Chapter 3 (see page 53), I explained that vegetable salads are a great way to end a fast because the fiber in veggies acts like a broom to sweep the intestinal tract clean. Fruits are also rich in fiber and have the advantage of being quick to digest. Grains, beans, legumes, and nuts are also high on the list of fast-transit foods, although not as high as fruits and vegetables.

Smart Animal Design

On page 109, I mention that four-legged animals have straight colons, which help them more easily move waste products to the anus for elimination. A number of four-legged animals have other biological advantages as well, especially when it comes to eating, digesting, and excreting meat. Many have sharp teeth that are designed to bite and tear flesh. Moreover, their digestive tract produces very powerful acids and enzymes that help digest meat more completely. Add in a short, straight colon—which has no "corners" and turns, like ours— and it's easy to understand why waste matter exits their bodies quickly and efficiently.

Another dietary component that aids bowel health and function is fluid, especially water. When you drink adequate fluids that keep the body properly hydrated, stool tends to be softer and easier to pass. When your body is dehydrated due to insufficient fluid intake or the consumption of dehydrating caffeinated beverages, the colon is forced to pull water from the stool, causing it to be hard and lumpy.

Do any foods actually slow the movement of waste through the body? Meat and dairy are more difficult for the body to digest, and when they pass into the colon, the food sometimes hasn't been completely broken down. This is precisely why heavy meat and dairy eaters tend to have more health problems as a whole. Fewer nutrients are absorbed into the body, and the food tends to sit in the colon longer as it breaks down. This can cause the food to putrefy in the "storage tank" of the colon, bringing on toxicity, which in turn can lead to health disorders. Note, too, that meat, dairy, and eggs contain no fiber, the helpful substance that speeds transit time.

While too much dairy can be harmful to your health, it is important to understand that certain dairy products, when used in moderation, can actually *improve* bowel health. To understand this, consider the fact that a healthy colon contains "friendly" bacteria, which helps the body fight off bacterial infections.

To help maintain a ready supply of this bacteria in the body, it's important to eat foods that actually contain a dose of these organisms. Foods such as yogurt, kefir, unprocessed cheese, and raw unpasteurized milk (preferably goat products) all fit the bill. Just be sure to enjoy these dairy products no more than three times a week, as they can form excess mucus and be a little more troublesome to pass through the colon. For a dairy-free dose of friendly bacteria, try natural sauerkraut. If none of these bacteria-promoting foods appeal to you, I suggest taking a friendly bacteria supplement called a probiotic, which is simply good, healthful bacteria in capsule, powder, or liquid form. Just remember that food is always infinitely preferable to supplements, and that probiotic products should be taken only when, for some reason, you do not wish to consume foods that include friendly bacteria, or when antibiotics are being used. (See the "Antibiotics" inset on page 112 for more information.)

Using Massage to Maintain Colon Health

In Chapter 1, I recommended that when you take a shower, you use massage to maintain the health of your lymphatic system. (See page 17.) This massage actually has a dual purpose, because it also enhances the health of the colon.

To understand the value of massage, you need to know a little about the ileocecal valve. This valve is actually a ring of muscle located at the junction of the small and large intestines (colon), to the right of the belly button. The purpose of this structure is to open up and allow the waste products in the small intestine to move into the colon, and then snap shut. It is intended to be a one-way valve. If the valve is "stuck" open, the waste products—including toxins—can flow from the colon back into the small intestine. If the valve is "stuck" closed, the waste products cannot flow into the colon but remain in the small intestine, creating another toxic situation. Maybe you have heard of the term "leaky gut." Problems with the workings of the ileocecal valve can actually cause the intestinal lining to become more permeable, leading to leaky gut syndrome, which is thought to play a part in inflammatory bowel disease, chronic fatigue syndrome, and several other disorders.

Journal Report

The Journal of Clinical Investigation confirmed, "Large bowel cancer is related to several factors. Among them, high dietary intake of animal fat, the presence in the colon of relatively high levels of bile acids, specific patterns of intestinal microflora, slow transit time through the gut, and low stool weights."[1] I know I don't want that.

Antibiotics

An antibiotic is a substance that is used to kill or inhibit the growth of "bad" bacteria—bacteria that is causing infection in the body. Unfortunately, antibiotics are indiscriminate in their targeting of bacteria, and kill the good organisms as well as the bad. Because good bacteria helps keep bad microorganisms in check, the body becomes more vulnerable to attack when friendly bacteria are eliminated. An article published in *Pediatrics* stated, "One cannot divorce the undesirable effects of antibiotics from the beneficial ones, and in this light, therapy becomes a calculated risk. If the probable discomfort or dangers outweigh the probable advantages, the cure may be worse than the disease, and one is then dealing with true iatrogenic disease [disease caused by treatment]."[2]

Rather than relying on antibiotics, I prefer to nourish my body's friendly bacteria. But if you must take antibiotics to control an infection, be sure to eat yogurt and other foods that provide beneficial bacteria, or to use probiotic supplements during the course of therapy. (See the discussion on page 111.) This will give your good bacteria the boost they need to keep your body in balance.

When you perform lymphatic self-massage, you will massage the valve and help it to work properly. If your valve is currently locked in an open position, the massage will help it close. If it is currently locked in a closed position, the massage will allow it to open. One of the first things I did for each of my patients was to make sure that the ileocecal valve was functioning properly. A well-functioning valve helps ensure proper absorption of nutrients and excretion of all wastes, including the toxic substances that can lead to ill health.

Treating Constipation

Earlier in this chapter, I explained steps you can take to help prevent a sluggish bowel without the use of artificial stimulants. But what can you do to relieve constipation when it is already a problem?

If you are currently suffering from constipation, I suggest that twice a day, you mix a tablespoon of flaxseed or olive oil in a glass of fresh juice, and drink it down. This will lubricate your colon and facilitate elimination. Another option is to mix a tablespoon of aloe vera juice in your homemade beverage. If you also include vegetables in your diet, preferably in the form of a daily salad, your bowels should soon function normally again.

Robert, a patient in his mid-forties, was a former high school athlete and proud of it. But he wasn't as active as he had once been, and over the years, he had gained a lot of weight. With his high school reunion coming in a few weeks, Robert shared his plan to quickly shed those unwanted pounds so that he could look like he had in his heyday. Robert was going to cut out all fruits, grains, dairy, oils, and sweets, and eat nothing but meat and some vegetables. I told Robert that although his plan to lose weight was noble, it was flawed because the high-protein diet would put his body under a great deal of strain. Over the years, many of my patients had lost weight on high-protein diets, but at a steep cost. All that protein had overburdened their bodies, resulting in a host of health problems, including intense lower-back pain. But Robert was undaunted by my warnings. He had made up his mind that high-protein was the way to go.

Robert proceeded on his "diet" and it worked! He lost quite a bit of weight, and six weeks later, he called to congratulate himself on his accomplishment. I commended him and wished him all the best, but again suggested that he change his dietary regimen. He said, "Hey, there is no stopping me now, I am on a roll."

Well, unfortunately, Robert was stopped. Two months later, he came to the clinic with intense back pain. I realized that he had ingested far too much meat, and that his colon, which was filled with partially digested food, and his kidneys, which had to filter out all that excess protein, were screaming for him to stop! After treating Robert for his pain, I put him on a supervised fast for a couple of days. Once he was feeling better, I shared my advice for a healthy lifestyle. Soon, he began to drink only clean water, eat clean foods, follow a once-a-week fast, exercise, and made sure he had a bowel movement every day, as well as integrating other healthful practices into his life. Eventually, his weight was right where he wanted it to be. It took some time before it got there, but Robert had learned that a healthy, pain-free lifestyle was every bit as important as a desirable weight.

HAND WASHING

While we're on the subject of bowel health, it is important to discuss a related subject—the need to wash your hands after "cleaning up" from a bowel movement. The waste product that is stored in the colon is far more toxic than the waste product that is stored in the bladder. While it's healthy to wash your hands after using the bathroom for any reason, it is *vital* to clean them after moving your bowels because of the bacteria and other toxic substances found in feces. You should also wash away any fecal matter that gets on your hands when changing a baby's diaper.

Eliminating a Narrowed Colon

When food doesn't get completely broken down, as is often the case with diets that are high in meat, waste products can build up on the colon walls, causing the organ to get increasingly narrow over time. Switching to a high-vegetable diet and drinking a tablespoon of olive oil or another natural lubricant in a glass of fresh juice can eliminate this problem.

Remember that any substance which lands on your hands—whether bacteria or other toxins—will be transported to your nose, mouth, or eyes the moment you touch your face. From there, the toxins can quickly get into your body, where they can cause a range of problems. That's why it's so important to wash your hands after going to the bathroom, before eating, and every so often throughout the day. (Your hands pick up germs wherever you go.) It is also a good idea to get in the habit of keeping your hands away from your face.

CONCLUSION

Ideally, the number of daily bowel movements you have will match the number of daily meals you eat. Even though you may not achieve this, I implore you to have a bowel movement *at least once a day.* If the day goes by without this occurring, make it a point to go into the bathroom and stay there until your colon has been emptied. You don't want the day's food to sit in your colon for several more hours while you sleep. If it does, instead of detoxifying, repairing, and rebuilding your body during the night, you will add toxins to your system.

Fortunately, there's a lot you can do to ensure healthy elimination. Good food, pure water, exercise, and self-massage—as well as the many other lifestyle components recommended in this book—will optimize the function of your digestive system and greatly aid the elimination process.

Whew! I'm glad I've finished covering this subject. You are doing a great job and have completed step eight on the road to remarkable health.

Remember, Health is Wealth!

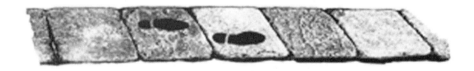

9. The Mind

Is it all in your head?

In Chapter 7, I addressed the importance of spending a few minutes alone each night so that you can review your day or perhaps spend some time in prayer. This quiet time of reflection helps to calm and detoxify your mind, your emotions, and even your soul. But are there things you can do to not only detoxify your mind, but also repair and rebuild it? The answer is yes, there is *plenty* you can do—and the benefits will include not only greater mental well-being, but also greater overall health. An article published in the *Journal of Clinical Endocrinology & Metabolism* suggested, "A healthy mind will define a healthy body, and vice-versa."[1] This chapter will look at some of the steps you can take to make your mind healthy and sound.

STARTING THE DAY

The way in which you start your day will help set the tone and rhythm of your life, so instead of waking up to the electronic sounds of a radio or the jarring buzz of an alarm clock, try awakening naturally or using a wake-up light. Similarly, instead of turning on the TV first thing in the morning, consider having a quality conversation with your loved ones, or playing positive and uplifting music that your whole family can benefit from and enjoy.

As you learned in Chapter 4, I also suggest that each morning you go for a short walk outside, preferably in the sunshine, followed by a short exercise routine. Once your exercises have been completed, take a therapeutic shower, preferably with a filtered showerhead so that your body comes in contact with the cleanest water possible. Following the instructions that begin on page 17, massage your lymphatic glands and use a loofah sponge to remove dead skin cells and help your body detoxify. For the last minute or so, run cool water to stimulate your circulatory system. This routine will add only a couple of minutes to your shower time, but will greatly improve your feeling of health and well-being.

Always set aside a few minutes to have a healthy breakfast, such as freshly made fruit juice and natural granola cereal, toast or bagel with dairy butter or nut butter, and perhaps an egg. I like to boil several eggs on the weekend and keep them in the refrigerator so that I have ready access to prepared eggs all week. I don't concern myself at all with the cholesterol hype about eggs. Your body is designed to easily digest and absorb the nutrients contained in the egg just fine, thank you. In fact, organic free-range eggs are one of the healthiest foods you and your family can eat. (See page 27 of Chapter 2 for more information about the benefits of eggs.)

If you drive or otherwise commute to work, try to maintain your positive mood as you travel to your job. For many people, the morning commute provides more time in which they can reflect and mentally prepare themselves for the upcoming day.

FRANK—A CASE STUDY

Frank came to my clinic complaining of headaches. He said that he would get a headache every day starting around noon, and the headache would increase in intensity as the day progressed until it got to be quite painful by evening. Frank mentioned he had a hard time falling asleep at night because of his consistent headaches.

I noticed how tired Frank looked, and could easily tell that he wasn't getting a whole lot of sleep. Frank went on to explain that he experienced a good deal of stress at work and that his boss put undue pressure on him. Frank was a salesman, and he was expected to satisfy a monthly quota of sales. Since he was a supervisor as well, he also had to make sure that other employees reached their quotas. The stress was taking its toll not just on Frank, but also on his wife and children.

After my examination, I told Frank that he was getting headaches because his mind never relaxed, but was always filled with the pressures of work. Mentally, Frank never really left the office even when he went home to his family. I explained that he needed to take time every night to detoxify his mind, and suggested that he put up a page-a-day calendar in his office. Each evening, as he turned off the lights and prepared to go home, he should simply tear off that day's calendar page and throw it away to signify that he had done all he could do, and now the workday was over. He should then go home and enjoy his family. Before he went to bed at night, he might even spend some time alone giving thanks to God for blessing him with family, friends, and yes, even work.

Frank followed this advice, and his headaches went away. By letting go of each workday before returning home, he allowed his mind to relax and refocus on other important areas of his life, including his wife and children.

ENDING THE DAY

As already discussed, it's important to spend some quiet time alone before bed-time. Review your day and calm your mind so that it is ready for sleep. I often take the opportunity to do some positive reading during this quiet time. Each week, I choose reading material that will inspire me to be a better husband, father, teacher, coworker, leader, and friend. This reading can come from a num-ber of positive sources. Many religious books are inspirational and offer words of wisdom and practical help. Many secular books are also well worth reading.

Over the years, I have treated countless patients who simply made up their minds that they were going to get well. One of the first steps on their journey of attaining greater health was to repair and rebuild their mind, emotions, social well-being, and soul with affirming activities. An important part of this process was to spend a few minutes each evening in a quiet, calm, and positive manner so that they could put their cares aside and benefit from a night of deep, untrou-bled sleep.

FINDING A PURPOSE IN LIFE

Everyone needs to find a purpose in life—a reason to get out of bed in the morn-ing. One great reason to get up and get going is that you are going to spend part of your day helping someone else. There is always someone who would benefit from the time you can spend with her, the knowledge you can share with her, or the money you can contribute to assist her. Helping others is not just a worthy pursuit, but also a way to make you feel good about yourself. Good thoughts and deeds are like boomerangs in that they tend to come back to you. The more you give to others, the more likely that you will be on the receiving end of pos-itive actions and attitudes. Moreover, when you share knowledge with some-one, you generally learn from that person. It has also been my experience that when you spend time with others, you tend to organize your own time more efficiently so that you can get more accomplished.

Of course, the reason for giving should not be that you will receive some-thing in return. Yet research has shown that the benefits of helping others are very real. An article in the *International Journal of Behavioral Medicine* stated, "Current research does indeed show a strong association between kindly emo-tions, helping behavior, or both, on one hand, and well-being, health, and longevity, on the other." The article continued, "It is already well established that compassion, love, and social support have health benefits for recipients. . . Volunteer behavior that is motivated by concern for the welfare of the other, rather than by anticipation of rewards, will improve morale, self-esteem, posi-tive affect and well-being."[2]

Treating Addictions

If you are in the throws of addiction or feel that you are on the road to substance abuse, please seek help. Whether your addiction is of a physical, psychological, social, or emotional form—or a combination of all four—the fact is that you *can* overcome your habit and live a healthier life. Try to find a professional or a clinic that will not only treat your symptoms, but also get to the cause of your addiction and consider your whole being throughout the treatment process.

One practice that can be helpful in the treatment of addiction is fasting. A supervised fast of up to a week in length can do wonders to break an unhealthy habit. I mentioned in the fasting chapter that a twenty-four-hour-a-week fast is sufficient for most people. However, extended fasts along with counseling have an important place in the treatment of addiction, as they rid the body of the toxins that can contribute to substance abuse. (I also find acupuncture helpful in treating this problem.) Usually, after twenty-four hours of taking in only water, you should switch to juices for the remainder of the fast. After this, it is helpful to follow a diet of organic foods and pure water along with a lifestyle that includes gentle rhythmic exercise, sunshine, adequate rest, proper posture, and a continual recharging of the mind through contact with positive people and inspirational books, movies, and music.

KEEPING YOUR MIND YOUNG AND HEALTHY

Most people who are "mature"—who are no longer kids, in other words—are rightfully concerned about keeping their brains in good working order. One way to maintain brain health is to keep the body healthy through exercise, proper nutrition, and the other lifestyle habits discussed within this book. Another way is to keep learning.

Learning—through education, through work experience, or through hobbies and other personal pursuits—has benefits far beyond the acquisition of knowledge. It's true that by gaining more information and skills, you can have a more rewarding and enjoyable life. But beyond that, the mind continually wants and needs to be stimulated in a positive way. Studies have shown that by constantly learning new things and challenging your mind through crossword puzzles and other "brain teasers," you will keep your mind healthy, sharp, and alert for many more years. Remember: You're never too old to learn something.

SHIRLEY—A CASE STUDY

Shirley was a senior who at the young age of ninety-two, would bring her neighbor's daughter—a young woman of thirty-five—to my clinic for treatment. Yes, Shirley was still driving quite well, thank you. I also noticed that as Shirley sat in the waiting room, she was never idle, but always occupied herself by doing a crossword puzzle, reading a book, or perusing the daily newspaper.

One evening, as I was finishing up for the day, I got a chance to visit with Shirley. I was amazed by how healthy she looked not only for a ninety-two-year-old woman, but for a person of any age. I just had to know her "secret" to staying healthy and vibrant. She said, "Young man, the 'secret' to staying young is to keep your mind active!" I had to smile. She went on to say that throughout her lifetime, she had followed many of the same recommendations for a healthy life that I had been sharing with her neighbor's daughter. As Shirley said, "They just make sense."

CONCLUSION

I've said it before and I'll say it again: I don't want to simply *hope* that I won't suffer from ill health. I want to take charge of my life and do everything necessary to remain healthy and active. You now know that this includes taking proper care of your mind. Just as you must detoxify, repair, and rebuild your body, you must detoxify, repair, and rebuild your mind by following healthy daily habits, spending time with uplifting people, reading inspirational books, helping others, and continuing to develop and use that important organ called the brain. A sound mind is an essential part of overall health. What the mind can conceive the body can achieve!

Congratulations: You have completed step nine on your road to excellent health.

Remember, Health is Wealth!

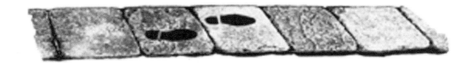

10. Building an Emotionally Satisfying Family Life

It all begins in the home.

As discussed in earlier chapters, good health involves a number of different components, including emotional well-being. While not everyone needs a family to be emotionally well, the fact is that a dysfunctional family makes it difficult if not impossible to have a satisfying emotional life, while a family in which members are cooperative and happy provides each individual with invaluable support and a sound foundation for a contented life.

Of course, a happy, well-functioning family is like a beautiful garden—it does not sprout up on its own. Instead, it needs a basic understanding of certain principles, a good deal of tender loving care, and lots of plain old-fashioned hard work. That's what this chapter is all about. It provides the simple guidelines needed to restore balance to a family and maintain an environment in which everyone can enjoy excellent emotional health.

MEETING A CHILD'S FOUR BASIC NEEDS

Every parent knows about the challenges of raising healthy, well-adjusted children. But over the years, I have found that if you meet four basic needs, you will go a long way toward helping your child enjoy emotional health.

The first of a child's needs is that for stability and routine. You should begin filling this need when your child is in early infancy by making sure that his diaper is changed regularly, that he is fed on a consistent schedule, and that he sleeps and plays at the same times each day. I thoroughly endorse a live-life-by-the-clock approach and a twenty-four-hour circle of life. Children actually yearn for routine and thrive on a consistent schedule. (For more information on this, see page 98 of Chapter 7.) Moreover, routine—which includes regular family meals and sleep times—promotes bonding between family members and supports physical well-being. An article in the *Occupation, Participation and Health* journal stated, "Family routines and rituals offer the opportunity to fully participate in family health."[1]

ELIZABETH—A CASE STUDY

Elizabeth was a married mother of two small children, and also worked outside the home. She was a very nice person, but always seemed disorganized and frazzled. She initially came to my clinic to ask for prenatal advice, as she was pregnant with her third child. I felt that congratulations were in order, but that was not what Elizabeth wanted to hear because she was already overwhelmed by her family of four. She said that her children didn't listen to her, her husband didn't respect her, and she didn't much care for her job, either. She already regretted missed opportunities, and now she was expecting another baby! It soon became clear to me that although Elizabeth was, on the surface, asking for prenatal advice, she was really crying out for guidance that would allow her to create a happier, healthier family.

I decided to give Elizabeth advice that had worked in my life and the lives of my patients. I began by telling her about the importance of filling a child's requirements for stability, security, love, and understanding of self-care. I also discussed the need to reinvigorate her marriage by doing all the "little things" that had originally made her relationship special—things like calling her husband in the middle of the day for no other reason than to say "Hi." Finally, I told the harried mother that although she felt that she had missed out on some opportunities, each day was a new beginning, and that it would be a far happier and more successful beginning if it included a central purpose, someone to love, and something to look forward to. (See the inset "Three Things You Need Each and Every Day" on page 125 for more information on these topics.) Elizabeth seemed to feel better after our conversation and was more than willing to put my advice into action.

Several months later, I ran into Elizabeth in the supermarket, and she looked like a different person. She said that her relationships had improved with both her children and her husband. Moreover, she was taking some college courses to further her career, and her boss was thrilled that she wanted to grow with the company. Elizabeth had been able to detoxify her emotions and had begun to repair and rebuild her emotional health. Soon after, she made an appointment to discuss ways in which she could further improve her well-being through clean water, clean food, fasting, exercise, sunlight, good posture, adequate rest, and the recharging of her mind. I am delighted to say that Elizabeth's efforts allowed her to vastly improve not only her own physical, mental, and emotional health, but also that of her children and spouse.

The second fundamental need of infants and children is security. By this I mean that the infant, and later the child, must be able to count on getting what he needs from his parents or other caregivers. He has to know that when he wakes up from sleep, someone will be there for him. He has to know that he will be fed. He has to know that when a parent promises to pick him up from school at a certain time, the parent will be there. He has to know that he can count on those who take care of him.

The third need is that for love. Children need to know that they are loved unconditionally, with no strings attached, and that their home is a safe haven. It is important to not simply assume that your child knows that you love him, but to express your love so that he has no doubts about your feelings. Several times a day, I tell my children how much I love them, how proud I am of them, and what a blessing they are to me and their mother. I also express my love through hugs and kisses—even when we're in a public setting. When my daughter is picked up from school, she gets a big hug and kiss. If you do not give your children the love that they need, they will seek it elsewhere.

Finally, a child needs you to teach him how to take care of his body, mind, emotions, social well-being, and soul. Again, if you do not provide your child with this important information, someone else will, and you may not approve of how or what he is being taught.

And So It Is Said

"If you have health, you probably will be happy, and if you have health and happiness, you have all the wealth you need, even if it is not all you want."
—ELBERT HUBBARD, WRITER, ARTIST, AND PHILOSOPHER

SETTING BOUNDARIES

Above, I discussed the four basic needs that must be met for every child. But it's also important to make your child aware of boundaries that should never be crossed without repercussions. My children know that they must never commit the three D's—disobedience, disrespect, and dishonesty. What happens if they do? They are given a punishment that fits the severity of the wrongdoing. For instance, they might be given a time out for a small failure to obey, have privileges taken away for an act of disrespect, or get a swat on the posterior for telling a lie. If the transgression is really severe, they might receive all three punishments.

It is important to be a fair but firm parent. Children must understand what the boundaries of their behavior are and what the punishment will be for crossing these boundaries. This means that you must be ready to carry out a punishment when it is warranted. I have seen many children lose respect for their parents when the child did something he knew he was not supposed to do, and the parent failed to follow up with discipline. As you probably know, children will at times cross boundaries just to see if their parents mean what they say and say what they mean.

Discipline should be a private matter. I have seen many parents embarrass and humiliate their children in public "to teach them a lesson." This is never a good idea. If my children transgress in public, I let them know which boundary has been crossed, and that a punishment will take place when we get home. Then I keep my promise. But I never allow myself to discipline my children in anger. Disciplining should be done out of love. If you find yourself fuming in anger over your child's actions, take some time to compose yourself before meting out punishment.

Once the punishment has been administered, I always cradle my children in my arms and tell them how much I love them. Yet I also make it clear that their poor behavior will not be tolerated and that if it happens again, they will be disciplined again. I always make sure that my children understand why they were punished, and even have them articulate their understanding of the boundary they crossed. I also explain why that boundary exists in the first place.

DEFINING EXPECTATIONS

Another important component of raising an emotionally healthy child is making your expectations for your child known. In my home, my children are given age-appropriate responsibilities as they mature and are expected to do their best at every endeavor they undertake. We do not want them taking a halfhearted approach to each activity, whether it is studying for an exam or practicing the piano before their next lesson. Of course, in order to set reasonable expectations for your children, you have to understand them so that you can get them involved in activities that are suited to them—activities that they will enjoy and at which they can succeed. This means spending quality time with your children, getting to know them on a very deep level, and helping them learn about you by sharing your life experiences, accomplishments, hopes, and dreams. You want to get to the point where when you look into your child's eyes, each of you knows what the other is thinking. This level of closeness will take some time, but your children—and your precious relationships with your children—are worth it.

MEETING YOUR SPOUSE'S NEEDS

It is vital to recognize that your spouse—not just your child—needs your love. When I worked with my patient Elizabeth (see the case study on page 121), I explained that love is not something that is demanded or taken from someone. It is something that is given freely.

If you are married, think back to how you felt on your wedding day. On that day, you were probably filled with love and respect for your partner. Well, love is like a beautiful garden, which needs tending not for one day only, but every day. Don't take your spouse for granted. Remember the little things you used to do when you were first together and return to doing them again, as if you were still courting. Send notes of love and phone your spouse just to say "Hello." Instead of demanding that your spouse perform certain tasks around the home, and then waiting angrily for him to do the vacuuming, pick the clothes up off the floor, or perform some other assigned duty, jump in and try to perform these tasks out of love. Once you start recreating the positive, caring atmosphere of your first days together, you will probably find that your spouse appreciates your gestures and is willing to become the person that you once married.

MAKING YOUR CORE VALUES CLEAR

I believe that in each home, there needs to be a set of core values—basic family philosophies and guidelines—that are printed out and perhaps posted on the wall. One of my values is that my wife is a gift from God, not my possession and not someone of whom I can make demands. Another is that I will treat my wife the way I treated her when we first started dating by showing her love, kindness, and respect at all times, and especially when the children are present. A third value is that I will continue to learn about and grow with my wife, which means that I will participate in the activities that she finds enjoyable—even ones I don't like, such as opera. It gives me real pleasure to share in her happiness. Plus, as one of my patients stated, "If mama ain't happy, ain't nobody happy." But my core values extend beyond the treatment of my wife to our treatment of the children. I also believe that my children are gifts from God and must be loved and nurtured.

Again, your core values should not be kept secret, but should be stated in a clear and plain way to the other members of your family. My values are printed on a framed certificate and hung on a wall of our home so that my children will read them from time to time, and will eventually acquire the knowledge needed to create their own happy, emotionally healthy families.

CONCLUSION

A happy, healthy family is one of the greatest gifts we can give to ourselves and the ones we love. It takes knowledge, attention, and daily work, but by meeting the basic needs of your children, your spouse, and yourself, you can create a

Three Things You Need
Each and Every Day

People who are discontented or bored with their daily existence cannot communicate a positive attitude to other people, whether those people are friends or family members.

One of the ways in which you can increase your level of happiness is to make sure that each day includes three important things: something meaningful to do, someone to love, and something to which you can look forward. For instance, if you find that you are not happy with the bulk of your day, it is time to find something that will be more meaningful to you, and then make the sacrifices necessary to reach your goal. You may, for example, have to downsize your home in order to finance the college courses that can lead to a more satisfying career.

Having someone to love can provide a purpose to your life, add to your joy during good times, and offer support in bad times. Remember, too, that you may be able to find great peace and happiness in your relationship with God. Personally, my greatest love is the love that I have with God.

Finally, you need something to which you can look forward, whether it is a short-term goal such as finding time to read a good book, or a long-term goal such as going on a vacation or working toward a promotion. This will help keep life interesting, increase your daily motivation, and encourage you to plan for the future. I am reminded of the saying, "Failing to plan is planning to fail."

positive environment that fosters emotional well-being in every family member, from the youngest to the oldest.

You have reached step ten on the road to achieving glorious health.

Remember, Health is Wealth!

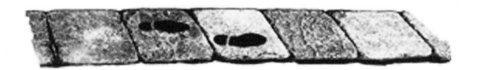

11. Social Relationships

People really do need people.

I was driving down the road the other day with the top down, wind blowing through my hair, music coming from my surround sound system, a long scarf flowing from my neck, and not a care in the world . . . maybe that was a movie I had just seen. I was listening to music, though. The radio was playing a popular song about a person who didn't need or want a friend or family to lean on, and was facing the cold, brutal world all by her lonesome. I reflected that this song not only was sad, but also presented an unhealthy me-against-the-world concept. People who are isolated, without support from others, tend to experience ill health along with an obvious lack of social well-being. We all need other people, whether it's a family of spouse and children, or simply good friends.

I know of several people who do not like to interact with others for fear of being hurt by them. They had their feelings injured at one time in their life, and retreated into their shell like a turtle that will not come out until it is safe. If you've been hurt in the past, or if you're simply shy or uncertain around other people, this chapter was designed to help you reach out with ease and success. It begins by briefly exploring our basic social nature, and then provides practical advice for creating and maintaining healthy, lasting relationships.

WE ARE SOCIAL BEINGS

Remember when you were a small child in kindergarten (for some of us that may take a bit of remembering), and most of the kids on the playground seemed to get along and play with one another? It's natural for kids to want to join in group play and be included in the fun. This is important, because it is through games and other group activities that children begin to learn how to get along with one another, how to share, and how to form friendships.

Eventually you grew up—not just physically, but also emotionally, mentally, and socially—and along the way, it is probable that you stopped joining in

Journal Report

The *Journal of Personality and Social Psychology* published an article that suggested, "Early social competence, in turn, should predict stronger related secure-based friendships during adolescence and expression of less negative versus positive emotions in adult's romantic relationships."[1] That makes sense to me.

playground games with your peers. Hopefully, though, you interact with friends in different ways. Yet not everyone does. So many people go through life alone, just trying to pay the bills and get through each day. They have lost their sense of social play. I realize that some people enjoy time alone more than others, and that there are times when everyone wants and needs to be alone, but throughout my years of treating patients, I noticed that the people who have the most joy and fun in their lives, as well as the greatest physical health, are those who share their lives with others. People who spend most of their time alone become filled with the toxins that can lead to disease and degeneration.

A few years ago, when watching the Olympics on TV, I saw the winner of a race cross the finish line as a stadium full of people clapped and cheered. He won the gold medal. A few days later, a reporter congratulated the athlete on his victory and asked how he felt about winning the award. To everyone's astonishment, he said he felt a little unfulfilled because he had no one with whom he could share his triumph. He went on to explain that he had spent so many years in training that he had never taken the time to cultivate relationships with other people. His life revolved around eating, sleeping, and training, with very little room for anything else. After the Olympics, he had gone home to an empty house and had simply placed his medal in a sock drawer. What would have made his victory more significant to him? People.

DEVELOPING SOCIAL RELATIONSHIPS

Some lucky individuals seem to be born with "people skills" and find it easy to establish and maintain social relationships. Some people find making friends a bit more challenging. But the process of making and keeping friends and romantic attachments is not a secret and is not all that difficult, either. In fact, anyone can make friends by opening themselves up to others and following a few simple guidelines. The tips presented on page 129 should help.

RUSSELL—A CASE STUDY

My new patient, Russell, was a man in his mid-twenties. I came bounding into the examination room with my hand outstretched to greet him by name, and he stared at me with a perplexed look on his face. I realized that he did not want to shake hands with a stranger. I didn't think I was strange, but I guess to him, I was a stranger. As we began reviewing his symptom survey form, it became obvious that he was very uncomfortable, and I finally realized that he was especially uneasy around my nurse assistant. I made eye contact with my assistant and indicated that she should kindly excuse herself from the room. Soon, Russell began to relax. We once again started to discuss his symptoms, but I knew it would just be a matter of minutes before he explained what was really bothering him.

Russell told me that he was once in a loving relationship for five years when his girlfriend—whom he had hoped to marry—said, "Russell, I want to date someone else." Russell was hurt by this comment, but being a kind and understanding man, he told her that he would wait for her to come back to him. He had waited for five years and still hadn't heard from her. During that time, he was afraid to talk to a member of the opposite sex for fear of rejection. He also had few male friends and no one with whom he could talk about his feelings. Russell longed for a relationship with a woman, but had chosen the safety of isolation instead.

I told Russell that he needed to get out of his turtle shell. Yes, he had been hurt, and no one likes to be hurt, but he needed to open up and create healthy social relationships. I then provided Russell with basic information about striking up conversations and building friendships, whether with a romantic partner or a platonic friend. (See pages 129 to 130 for more information on this.) Finally, I treated Russell for the physical symptoms that had motivated him to visit my clinic in the first place. But that day, he left my office with far more than he had hoped to get from his appointment.

About six months later, Russell called to say that he had met a lovely lady at church. He had struck up a conversation, she was interested, and the relationship had begun to grow. Within a year, I received an invitation to Russell's wedding, which I was delighted to attend. Eventually, Russell and his new wife even visited my clinic for help with her health problems, and she began a successful program that included clean water, clean food, a weekly fast, and the other lifestyle components discussed in this book. Just as important, she developed rewarding relationships with friends and family members who made her life fuller, happier, and healthier.

❏ **Be aware of your good qualities.** Before you go out into the world to meet new people, boost your self-esteem by thinking about your good qualities—things about you that other people would find attractive. Can't think of any good qualities? Well, are you honest and hard-working? Do you love children? Do you take good care of your pets? These are all pluses and are not true of everyone. Also think about the activities that you enjoy and would like to share with others. Perhaps you love watching old movies, reading mystery stories, going to the zoo, or cooking. These interests will not only make you an appealing person, but also give you something to talk about when you meet someone new.

❏ **Start the conversation off with a compliment.** This is especially helpful if you're meeting someone of the opposite sex, but really, compliments are always welcome and so easy to do. I really do like the old saying, "If you can't say something nice, don't say anything at all." When I advised my patient Russell (see the case study on page 128), I told him to start a conversation with a woman by complimenting what she is wearing. If you are just trying to strike up a friendship, you can compliment the other person's taste regarding her car or another "neutral" topic.

❏ **Give people an opportunity to talk about themselves**. Most people love to talk about themselves and value a companion who actively listens to them. So show interest in other people and ask questions that will allow them to talk about themselves. For instance, if you are chatting with someone at a party, you might ask, "Do you like the food?" or "What brings you to this gathering?" The more you show an interest in other people, the more they will appreciate you and want to learn more about you.

❏ **Be an attentive listener.** When other people are talking, don't look down, off into the distance, at your watch, or at the people milling around you. Instead, look directly at the speaker, smile when appropriate, and occasionally ask a question or make an appropriate comment—without taking over the conversation and focusing it on yourself. This will demonstrate that you are truly interested in what the other person has to say.

❏ **Try to find something that you have in common with the other person.** The more you have in common with someone, the easier it will be to build a relationship with that person. Once you find common ground—whether it is the love of golf, an interest in gardening, or just the fact that you both take the train to work—you can get along with just about anyone, even a rival. In time, you will be able to build a relationship, which can be casual or serious, platonic or romantic. But it all starts with breaking the ice and communicating.

❏ **Continue to pay compliments and show respect for the other person over time.** How many relationships have already come and gone in your life? The reason that so many relationships dissolve is either that the people never bothered to appreciate each other's good qualities to begin with, or that they stopped complimenting and actively listening to one another over time. People are drawn to each other through likeability, respect, and admiration. This is what causes them to stop and learn more about the other individual. But it's not enough to show respect and admiration at the beginning of a relationship; you have to continue to treat the other person well throughout your time together. Say positive things. Show interest in your companion's opinions and interests. Make it clear that you value the other individual. This will cause your relationship, whether it's a friendship or a romance, to take root and flourish.

❏ **Don't try to change the other person.** Many people enter relationships in the hope that they will be able to mold the other person into what they want her to be. They wish that the other individual was neater, slimmer, more athletic, more ambitious, or more social. Generally speaking, people will change only if they want to change, and your attempts to transform your friend or partner into something else will not only fail, but also doom the relationship itself to failure.

CONCLUSION

Healthy social relationships are gifts beyond measure. And fortunately, if you follow a few guidelines, you can successfully make a friend or even start a romance. You don't have to be an island of one.

In this chapter, you've learned some of the basics of establishing and nourishing good relationships. Start off by paying a compliment, show your interest in the other person, and find common ground. It is during this time of getting to know one another that a relationship will begin to develop. Some people will turn into casual acquaintances, while others will become lifelong friends or even develop into romantic partners.

Congratulations, you have just completed step eleven on the road to exuberant health. Remember Health is Wealth!

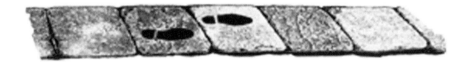

12. The Soul

Creating a loving relationship with God.

Now, I know what you're thinking: If you wanted to hear a sermon, you would have gone to church, temple, or another house of worship. Don't worry, though. I won't be preaching today. I'll just be offering tips that can help you find your way to a better relationship with God.

I grew up in church. I was baptized as an infant and confirmed as a teenager. I thought that I knew all about God and felt that I had been given a road map to follow for the health of my soul. But as I got older, I realized that I didn't really know God at all, at least not on a personal level, and that my map was *man's* idea of what it took to have a healthy soul, not God's. In short, I had a road map but no direction. Which way should I go? What road should I take throughout my life? And how would I find God, who seemed so far away?

I realize now that my feelings as a young adult were not unique to me. So many people receive religious guidance as children and teenagers, but still have a restless soul that feels empty. Despite the instruction, rituals, and celebrations that were part of their religious upbringing, they are confused and unsure what to believe. I was fortunate in that I found the road that I was meant to travel and developed a rewarding relationship with God. The result was not only greater happiness, but also a healthy soul that has contributed to my overall health. The remainder of this chapter will guide you, too, in nourishing your soul so that this important aspect of your life contributes to your well-being.

DEVELOPING YOUR RELATIONSHIP WITH GOD

For most people, the absence of a relationship with God results in a feeling of restlessness and allows the pollutants of the world to settle into the soul so there is no inner peace. In a world that is so full of negativity, you need to be vigilant about detoxifying, repairing, and rebuilding your soul.

CARL—A CASE STUDY

Carl, a man in his mid-thirties, was sitting in my clinic one afternoon, waiting for his friend to finish his treatment. I always knew when Carl arrived at my clinic because I could hear him in the lobby, slapping people on the back and exclaiming about what a glorious day it was. Carl seemed to have life all figured out. He was gregarious and appeared to be without a care in the world. I was therefore surprised one afternoon when Carl asked if he could speak to me. I had a roomful of patients waiting for me, but I could see in Carl's eyes that he really wanted and needed to talk.

As it turned out, despite Carl's life-of-the-party image, he felt alone. His outgoing behavior was just his way of hiding his loneliness. When the party was over, he went home to an empty house. He had no family and no close friendships. He had no relationship with God because he felt unworthy of being loved. Carl's whole life was one of pretense and superficiality.

I felt that Carl's greatest problem was that he was missing the important ability to love someone much greater than himself and to feel that love returned. In other words, he lacked a loving relationship with God and was in deep need of healthcare for the soul. I urged Carl to spend time alone with God through prayer so that he could feel his divine energy. I also counseled him to listen to uplifting radio programs and read inspirational books, including the Scriptures. (For more information on developing a relationship with God, see the discussion that begins on page 131.)

A few weeks later, Carl asked to speak to me again. He said that he had implemented my suggestions for improving the health of his soul, and they had changed his life. I told him that it was God who had changed him—that my suggestions had simply helped Carl start the process of healing his soul. Later, Carl made a real appointment, and I mapped out a plan for his healthcare that included pure water, clean food, exercise, and the suggestions previously discussed in this book. Carl jumped in with both feet and enthusiastically traveled the road to physical, mental, emotional, and spiritual health. Over time, he not only developed a stronger relationship with God, but also established positive social bonds. Carl is a backslapper to this day, but is a healthy, happy, and contented person as well.

It's important to explore some of the very real benefits of developing a relationship with God. As mentioned above, it will nourish and satisfy your soul. It will also allow you to have a deeper and more loving relationship with other people, and when you truly love other people, you will not be aggravated by the little annoyances they can cause in your daily life. You will feel a forgiveness that will set your soul free and keep you from harboring the negative thoughts that can make your soul toxic. Remember that the only one who suffers from the resentment you feel is you. When you love and forgive others without bitterness or anger, you will experience true joy. And when you give others some of your time, knowledge, or resources, your happiness will be far greater than it is when you do something for yourself.

A love of God will also help build character and sustain you through bad times. Too often, people stray from their faith, but when life takes a negative turn, they blame God. It is at these times, though, that faith—which is born of a love of God—can provide inner strength and inner peace.

Perhaps you're intimidated by the prospect of talking to God, who may seem like a very distant being in a far-away place. But anyone can speak to him. You don't need to belong to a specific club or organization, and you don't have to be a perfect person. The key to a relationship with God is simply being willing to open up your soul to him.

In previous chapters, I suggested that each night, before going to bed, you make some quiet time for yourself. (See page 101 of Chapter 7.) This will create a great opportunity to open your soul to God, allow him into your heart, and spend some time with him. Try to feel the love that you have for God and that he has for you. If you believe in a greater being, enabling that love to flow into your soul will do wonders for you. It will let you know that there is indeed someone watching over you with care and concern.

Simply talk to God as if he were your best friend. Share with him all your hopes, dreams, and yes, even your fears and disappointments. At first, this may seem awkward or forced, but as you establish a daily habit of talking to God, you will become more comfortable in communicating your feelings and thoughts to him.

In addition to talking to God, I strongly recommend praying to him. Praying to God is the single greatest way to detoxify your soul. I have personally integrated five aspects of prayer into my life. First, I thank God for the blessings he has already bestowed on me, such as my family and friends. Second, I praise God and acknowledge his supreme power. Third, I ask God to forgive me for any negative thoughts I have had, any negative words I have spoken, and any negative actions I have taken against God or against someone else. Fourth, I ask God to bless others, and finally, I ask God for his continual blessings upon my life. These five aspects are helpful in detoxifying my soul and providing structure in my communication with God.

I want you to know that over time, I have deepened my relationship with God, and I didn't do it by going to church. My relationship continues to grow whenever I spend time alone with God, just has my love for my wife and children increases as I spend more time with them and get to understand them on a deeper level. Each day, for a few minutes, I talk and pray to God. It is through these daily communications that I have gotten to know God, just as you can get to know him by opening your own soul to him. This may take a little time, but as you develop a close communion with God, he will establish in you a divine energy flow. In Chapter 5, you read about the energy that God provides through the sun and Earth. This energy can stimulate and improve your physical and mental health. Why not also experience the energy that God provides for your spiritual health?

DAN—A CASE STUDY

Most of the case studies in this book share stories of people whom I treated in my clinic. Dan was not one of my patients, but nevertheless served as an inspiration in my life.

Dan was a man of stature in my town. The president of a well-respected company, he was also married and the proud father of three children. As you might expect, he had a more-than-adequate salary, and he and his family were able to live well.

I was introduced to Dan by a friend when we all attended a local convention. As I shook Dan's hand, I immediately sensed that he was a man of peace and contentment. So many people have an air of importance and seem to need to validate themselves in your eyes from the moment you meet them. Dan had no such air, and I found that I wanted to learn more about him. Fortunately, during the course of the convention, I got to know him better.

Dan told me that the reason for his contentment was his relationship with God. God's love made him feel worthy, which not only allowed Dan to love God back, but also enabled him to love others as well as himself. Dan is not the first person to realize that the love of God is unique and has a special effect on those who accept it. The Biblical Research Journal stated, "The study of the love of God, agape in its usage of that which originates with God, deals with a new kind of love."[1] Agape (pronounced ag-e-pee) is considered the highest and purest form of love—the self-sacrificing love that God gives to man. It is no wonder that it permits us to love ourselves and others without bitterness, resentment, or judgment.

Dan was taking care of his soul by spending time with God and learning to love him on a deeper level. It was clear that this relationship gave Dan the strength of character, emotional calm, and spiritual health that made him the happy and successful man he was.

CONCLUSION

Remember, this book is not about making changes for a day, but about establishing lasting changes that will increase your health and happiness for a lifetime. By following the recommendations discussed in this chapter, you will detoxify, repair, and rebuild your soul, just as the advice presented in earlier chapters can help you heal and develop your physical, mental, emotional, and social well-being. You will have a peace about you. You will experience inner joy and contentment. You will find a love that will fill your life with happiness and enable you to love others in a new and deeper way.

There are a lot of toxins in this world. Just turn on the radio or television or read the newspaper. I recommend that you begin detoxifying your soul by spending time talking and praying to God. I advise that you repair and rebuild your soul by reading positive books, watching and listening to uplifting movies and music, and keeping company with people who respect your faith and your commitment to God. You will then be well on the road to attaining and maintaining your health. You have just completed step twelve on the road to wonderful health.

Remember, Health is Wealth!

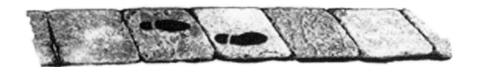

13. Preparing, Storing, and Eating Your Food

Getting the most out of your meals.

In Chapter 2, I presented guidelines for choosing good, healthy, clean foods. In the course of that chapter, I mentioned that it is best to eat food that is as close to its natural state as possible. Just the same, I don't think that you should eat your meat uncooked. You probably don't want to eat your eggs raw, either. You're more than likely to cook certain foods before eating them, and if you're concerned about following a healthy diet, you want to cook them in a way that preserves nutrients and doesn't impart toxins or any negative energy. You also want to store your food in a way that maintains its freshness. That's what this chapter is all about. In the following pages, you'll learn about choosing appliances and cookware, using the most wholesome cooking methods, storing foods wisely, and selecting the best dining utensils—everything you need to know to turn delicious, nourishing ingredients into equally enjoyable and beneficial meals. Finally, you'll discover a great way to make nutritious baby food that will be ready for your child on even the busiest day.

CHOOSING APPLIANCES AND COOKWARE

Good meals start not only with healthful ingredients, but also with good basic tools that help you get the most out of your foods. This includes both the appliances used to cook your food and the cookware in which the food is prepared.

Most conventional ovens offer a safe and dependable way to cook your meals. I prefer electric ovens and ranges to gas appliances because of a gas oven's potential to leak the gas being used and/or create a buildup of carbon monoxide. If you do use a gas oven, make sure to keep an exhaust fan going, and have your oven checked for leaks at least once a year. If speed is an important consideration, consider a convection oven, which is a conventional oven that uses a fan to circulate the heat throughout the cooking area. By moving the hot air quickly past the food, rather than just heating the food from below, this

Staying Young at Any Age

I do a lot of public speaking, and have always enjoyed talking at nursing homes. I love to meet the people there, but I am saddened as I see their health deteriorate week after week. The rewards can be great, though. Not long ago, I told an audience of nursing home seniors and staff members how natural, healthy lifestyle choices can be easily implemented at any age, whether you're a man or a woman, rich or poor. As long as you're willing to be proactive about your health, you can regain your health.

The lecture apparently woke up both the staff and the residents, because within a week, seniors were being wheeled out into the courtyard for sunlight; the menus included healthy dishes with plenty of raw fruits and vegetables; clean water was being used for drinking and cooking; a juice machine had been purchased; old pots and pans had been replaced with glass, ceramic, and stoneware; and shower filters were being installed. Everyone was encouraged to get in some walking, too. Residents and staff were even educated on the importance of rest, posture, and elimination. Many nurses had a newfound respect for living life like a clock, and the whole place seemed to buzz with healthy, positive energy. The next time I visit the senior home, I may see residents doing cannonball dives into the pool.

appliance cooks food more quickly than a conventional oven while using a lower temperature. This not only helps avoid burning, but can also help retain nutrients. Most significantly, unlike a microwave oven, a convection oven does not use electromagnetic radiation to heat or "zap" food.

As you may have gathered, one of the means of cooking food that I do *not* endorse is the microwave oven. This modern convenience has its consequences. Research has shown that microwaving damages many of the substances found in foods, makes nutrients less available to the body, and may contribute to the development of cancer. A study on the effects of microwaving on human milk demonstrated that the practice—a common means of thawing frozen milk in some nurseries—significantly decreases important anti-infective factors in breast milk. Scientists involved in the study stated, "Microwaving appears to be contraindicated at high temperatures, and questions regarding its safety exist even at low temperatures."[1] This is why I call microwaved food, *freak food*!

Finally, I'd like to address the option of grilling. Many people enjoy grilling, and I used to be one of those people because I liked the taste of grilled food.

Spicing It Up

When cooking a meal, most of us add herbs, spices, and that all-American favorite, salt. Herbs and spices are fine, and many contain valuable nutrients, but regular mined table salt contains inorganic compounds, which will put undue stress on your kidneys and harden your blood vessels. If you feel that you need to add a salty taste to food, try adding sea kelp or sea salt, and use in moderation. (See page 38 in Chapter 2 for more information on salt.)

However, one problem with grilled food, especially food that is cooked over a charcoal fire, is that it often absorbs a high amount of smoke. Consuming this food is actually comparable to breathing in second-hand cigarette smoke. Moreover, as an article published in the Oxford journal *Carcinogenesis* stated, grilling meats produces cancer-causing agents called HCAs (heterocyclic amines). The article stated, "Charred and black crusted materials on the surface of proteinaceous [protein-containing] foods, which are produced by contact with a naked flame, contain especially high levels of HCA's."[2] I do not recommend that you ever use a charcoal grill. Gas grills are better than charcoal grills, and electric grills are best, but all grilling can generate a carcinogenic substance called polycyclic aromatic hydrocarbon (PAH). For the healthiest results, grill your food at a lower temperature and/or farther from the heat source. This will result in the lowest level of PAHs.

Now that we've discussed the best ways to supply the basic heat used to cook foods, let's look at cookware. I believe that the best type of nonmetal cookware is made of pyroceramic glass, such as CorningWare; lead-free ceramic; or stoneware. These materials are good because they contain no man-made chemicals that can leach into foods during cooking and end up in your body.

Avoid all Teflon-coated and aluminum-based cookware. Teflon contains the toxin perfluorooctanoic acid (PFOA), which is a known carcinogen. Aluminum cookware, on the other hand, has been linked with Alzheimer's disease. The *Canadian Medical Association Journal* published an article stating, "Although the cause of Alzheimer's disease remains unknown, there is mounting evidence that implicates aluminum as a toxic environmental factor of considerable importance. . . . We hypothesize that a public health effort to resist human ingestion of aluminum would reduce the risk of this common chronic illness in the elderly."[3] I have been warning about this danger for years.

Although stainless steel is better than Teflon-coated or aluminum cookware, when used over high heat, stainless steel can leach inorganic minerals such as nickel and chromium into food. As discussed in Chapter 1, inorganic minerals cannot be processed by the body, and are therefore stored as a toxin if they are not eliminated. If you own stainless steel cookware, cook over low to medium heat.

CHOOSING COOKING METHODS

One of my general rules is that at every meal throughout the day, I eat some type of raw fruit or vegetable or drink some type of freshly made fruit or vegetable juice. The remaining dishes I enjoy cooked at low temperatures (cooked cereal, for instance) or cooked at higher temperatures (meat and eggs, for instance).

When foods are cooked, some of this nutritional value is retained, but much of it is just plain destroyed by heat. When foods are cooked at a temperature greater than 125°F, the nutrients start to diminish. Over 212°F, they diminish greatly. Cooking at high temperatures, in fact, eliminates many of the vitamins, minerals, amino acids, enzymes, and other nutrients found in food, leaving you with a pile of mostly empty calories. Many people literally starve themselves for nutrition while eating great quantities of poorly cooked foods. As long as you give your body vital nutrition through raw fruits and vegetables, it's okay to lose some of the nutrients through cooking. But it's important to choose the cooking methods that will deplete these nutrients as little as possible.

Enjoying Grains, Nuts, Seeds, and Legumes

Grains, nuts, seeds, and legumes can be eaten raw or sprouted. (To sprout them, leave them in water overnight, drain the water, soak overnight again, drain, and allow the food to dry for about forty-eight hours.) Most of the time, though, you will probably want to cook your grains and legumes, which may destroy some of the nutrients. This is fine as long as you include some raw vegetables and fruits in your daily diet.

The common methods of cooking, in order of personal preference, are: steaming, sautéing, boiling, broiling, baking, roasting, electric grilling, cooking in a wok, and frying. The last method on the list, frying, is my least favorite method of cooking. Due to the high heat involved, frying destroys nutrients more fully than any other method of preparing food with the exception of microwaving. I personally use most of the options listed above to prepare food, but I always include some raw vegetable or fruit with my meal to make sure I get nutrients in my diet.

NANCY—A CASE STUDY

My patient Nancy loved to cook. She would invite not only family and friends to dinner, but also people she had just met. Her kitchen was the heart of her home, and she prided herself on using only the most nutritious of ingredients when preparing meals for herself and her guests.

During one visit to the clinic, Nancy said that over the course of a few months, she had begun to feel tired and run-down. Although she was still cooking up a storm, she wasn't able to muster her usual enthusiasm for her favorite activity.

I asked Nancy how she cooked her food, and she explained that she usually fried or microwaved the food, and often used high heat. I explained that these cooking methods destroy nutrients and cause other harmful changes in food components. No wonder she was feeling so fatigued! Although she was buying nutrient-rich foods, by the time she had finished cooking them, the nutrients had been largely depleted.

I explained the need to eat raw fruits and vegetables as much as possible, and to cook foods through steaming or sautéing—methods known to retain nutrients. Nancy followed my suggestions and started to regain her energy and enthusiasm. She still cooked for everyone she knew, but now she maintained the high quality of her ingredients. Family and friends appreciated that the meals they enjoyed at Nancy's house were not only delicious, but also healthy.

CHOOSING DINNERWARE AND UTENSILS

When my family dines at home, we use plates, bowls, and other dinnerware made of lead-free ceramic, glass, or stoneware. No matter how long the food remains on these dishes, no harmful chemicals will leach into it. When we go on a picnic, I usually take our "real" plates and utensils along. Chlorine-free paper plates and cups are fine, too, but do avoid Styrofoam, which contains the toxins benzene and styrene and isn't exactly environmentally friendly, either.

Eating utensils made of stainless steel or even plastic are acceptable because contact between them and the food is brief. If you want a more natural choice, though, look for flatware made of bamboo. I recommend that you use wooden utensils when stirring foods during cooking, especially at higher temperatures.

STORING LEFTOVERS

I suggest enjoying your food as soon as it is prepared. In addition to being respectful to the person who cooked the meal, this will mean that you are getting maximum nutrients from your food. The great destroyers of your foods' vitamins, minerals, and other nutrients are air, light, and heat. The longer the food or beverage sits around, the more nutrients will be lost. If the food has been cooked, there is all the more reason to sit down and eat it. As you learned earlier in the chapter, cooking reduces the nutrients that remain in the food, so it's important to consume that food before more damage is done by time.

If some food is left over after a meal, or if you wish to pack your meal and take it to work or school, use containers made of glass, lead-free ceramic, or polyethylene plastic, or polypropylene plastic sandwich bags. These materials will not leach harmful chemicals into your food. Always cover the food and refrigerate it within an hour of preparation to slow bacterial growth. Do not, however, freeze meat once it has been cooked, as this practice can lead to food-borne illness.

Vegetable and fruit juices are especially perishable; they will begin to lose their nutrients as soon as they are made. If possible, drink your juices directly after preparation. If you have to store leftover juice, transfer the juice to a glass container, cover the container tightly to shut out air, and place it in the refrigerator. But try not to wait longer than a couple of hours before drinking the juice. The fresher it is, the healthier it will be. When you take the juice out of the refrigerator, let it warm up a bit before consuming it so that you put a warm liquid into your warm body. Cold liquids tend to stress the body, unless the body has been heated up (by exercise, for instance) and needs to be cooled down.

Food and Energy

As discussed earlier in the book, the Earth and sun emit positive electromagnetic energy. We absorb this healthy energy from the ground and the sunlight, as well as from clean food and pure water. Healthy individuals have their own positive vibrational energy field, as well.

When I treated patients, one of my goals was to rebalance and recharge their individual energy fields, and to help them avoid harmful negative energy, such as that emitted by microwave ovens. How can you recharge your own electromagnetic field? First, avoid a diet composed of only cooked foods, which will drain your energy instead of building it up. Include raw fruits and vegetables in every meal, either by eating whole fruit and vegetable salads or by drinking freshly made juices. Whenever possible, consume the seeds of the produce, too. Seeds, which contain the life force of the plant and provide a wide range of nutrients, will recharge your positive energy and help you look and feel revitalized.

Living in a Bubble

I do not recommend that you live in a bubble in which all food is organic and eaten raw at home, and no meals are enjoyed in restaurants or other people's homes. Simply try to do whatever is possible to make your life healthier. For example, it is fairly easy to replace your pots and pans with healthier types of cookware. You can also use more recipes that feature steaming and less that involve high heat. At your favorite restaurant, request that your food be prepared without use of a microwave oven. Remember that this book is not about sacrifice, but about replacing unhealthy habits with healthy ones. Maybe you will implement all of my suggestions, and maybe you will employ only a few. Whatever you do will be a positive step on the road to health.

If you often find yourself storing leftovers, I suggest that you buy a vacuum storage system. This system consists of see-through plastic containers and an air pump. The food is placed in a container, and the pump is attached to the container and used to pull out all of the air. Since air is one of the major villains in nutrient loss, this makes it possible to store food from four to five times longer in your refrigerator or freezer. These systems are relatively inexpensive and found in most supermarkets and houseware stores.

As a kid, I always disliked leftover food that was reheated the next day. I now realize that I probably could tell that my food had lost nutrition through storage and a second cooking. For this reason, I suggest that you eat your leftovers cold if possible. (Now, that doesn't mean that you should load up on yesterday's pizza!)

PREPARING BABY FOOD

I'd like to share with you a convenient way to prepare vegetables for your infants. Over the weekend, steam batches of clean organic carrots, yams, or broccoli until softened. Place the steamed vegetables in a large blender, add clean water, and process into a smooth paste.

Portion the vegetable paste out into clean ice cube trays, wrap the trays in freezer paper, and place them in the freezer. When the puréed vegetables are frozen, unwrap the trays, pop out the individual portions, and store them in freezer-safe plastic bags. Remember to seal the bags well so that the veggies are protected from air. When it's time to feed your infant, take one or two cubes out of the bag, place the food in a small glass container with a lid, and run warm water over it until the veggies are thawed. This will take only a couple of minutes. Now your infant has a warm vegetable pudding that is full of nutrients and easy to digest. I have tasted this vegetable "smoothie," and it really is quite delicious.

Sometimes, I take out the frozen veggie cubes the night before and place them in a small container in the refrigerator. By lunch the next day, the vegetables are ready to eat, either cool or briefly warmed under running water. This homemade food contains far more nutrients and is far purer than most commercial products.

When you prepare grains for your infant, cook the grains, place them in a blender with clean water, and process into a paste. Transfer the blended grains to covered glass bowls, and refrigerate until you are ready to serve the food to your baby. You will have nutritious, infant-ready cooked grains at your fingertips.

CONCLUSION

So many people ask me what they should eat, how they should cook their food, and even what type of dinnerware they should use at the table. Here is what I recommend: Eat a diet that includes vegetables and fruits at every meal; include grains, legumes, seeds, and nuts; consume smaller amounts of dairy and meat. Eat produce, nuts, and seeds raw whenever possible, and cook most other foods over relatively low heat in cookware made of glass, ceramic, or stoneware. Then serve your foods on glass, ceramic, and stoneware plates and bowls. Try to avoid leftovers, but if you do have some, wrap them well, store them in the refrigerator, and eat them cold or only lightly warmed. Remember that air, heat, and light will rob your food of nutrients.

I am confident that if you follow the recommendations outlined in this chapter, you will optimize the nutritional value of your meals. You have just completed step thirteen on the road to marvelous health.

Remember, Health is Wealth!!

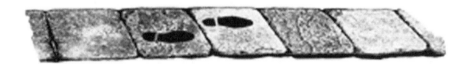

14. Beauty and Hygiene

Mirror, mirror on the wall . . .

O h, the never-ending quest for beauty. Just turn on your TV and you'll find commercials for potions that promise to deliver the "secret" of beauty and youthfulness. Unfortunately, many of these secrets can actually make your skin age faster than it would if you used no products at all. The vast majority of commercial products contain ingredients that you should not apply to your body. Earlier in the book, I mentioned that if a substance isn't good enough to put *in* the body, you should not put it *on* the body. This makes sense, because substances applied to the skin can readily be absorbed into the body.

My grandparents lived to a ripe old age, free of most of the health problems that are so common today. My grandmother was a beautiful woman both inside and out. I don't recall her using all the creams, potions, lotions, and oils that are now being touted. The best beauty "secrets" are really the simplest and least expensive, the way Nature intended.

Beauty's building blocks are the foods we eat, the water we drink, sunshine, fresh air, proper rest, frequent elimination, fasting, and exercise. If you follow the guidelines outlined in this book, your skin, hair, and nails will be healthy and strong, and you will be well on the way to looking great. The remainder of this chapter addresses other subjects you should know about as you strive for health and beauty.

A FEW WORDS ABOUT TOXINS

A number of toxic substances are commonly used in the cosmetic and hygiene products that you'll find in the average drugstore or department store. It is beyond the scope of this book to mention every potentially hazardous substance that may be included in beauty and personal-care preparations, but throughout this chapter, you'll find discussions of a number of them, including parabens, sodium lauryl sulfate, propylene glycol, triclosan, ascorbyl palmitate, and toluene. These and other chemicals can cause a toxic buildup on the skin and within the body, resulting in health problem ranging from skin rashes to a compromised immune system. You may wonder why all these and many other toxins are allowed to be used in our cosmetics. The Food and Drug Administration, or FDA, puts little effort into regulating the cosmetics industry, making the industry its own watchdog. And when an industry is allowed to regulate itself, we all know what can happen.

You should know that among the many toxins commonly used in personal care products are so-called *environmental estrogens,* which can mimic the effects of the hormone estrogen. Even at low levels, these substances can work together with the body's own hormones, increasing the risk of problems such as early puberty, infertility, breast cancer, early menopause, and early andropause (male menopause). Toxins in this group include the parabens (butylparaben, ethylparaben, and others), placental extracts, and benzophenones. These substances can be found in a variety of products, from shampoos to sunscreens and body lotions.

Just as this chapter does not name every potentially harmful substance, it does not mention the various symptoms that may be experienced if you use these products. Different people can have different responses when they come in contact with potentially harmful ingredients. Generally speaking, toxin-laden cosmetics react negatively with the skin at the point of use, but because some of the substance is also absorbed into the body, other problems can develop as the body tries to filter the toxins out. Moreover, the body may react not immediately after the product's use, but days, months, or even years later.

Dangers in the Cosmetics Aisle

An article published by the Environmental Working Group explained that many adolescent girls are being contaminated by the chemicals used in their cosmetics and body-care products. The article stated, "Studies link these chemicals to potential health effects including cancer and hormone disruption."[1] This points to yet another reason why young women are developing at a faster rate than earlier generations, and why hormone-related problems are occurring at younger ages. The same types of hormone-related problems are occurring in young boys.

Fortunately, it's really not necessary to know the name of every toxin used in beauty and personal-care products, nor do you have to know the possible symptoms. Just keep in mind a useful rule of thumb: If you can't pronounce the ingredient, or you have no idea what it is, you probably shouldn't use it and neither should any other member of your family. Select products that include recognizable natural ingredients—aloe vera, coconut oil, jojoba oil, and other wholesome substances—and you will rarely go wrong.

HAIR CARE

Most of us use hair-care products of some type, and some people use a collection of these beauty aids. For that reason, all of us need to know a little about selecting shampoos, conditioners, and similar items.

Shampoos and Conditioners

Sodium lauryl sulfate and sodium laureth sulfate are detergents and surfactants that are used in a range of products, including soaps and shampoos. These ingredients are even prominent in many so-called health food store products, which brings up another important truth: Just because something is in a health food store doesn't mean it's healthy. An article printed in the *Journal of Medical Sciences* stated, "It was concluded that Sodium Lauryl Sulfate is a skin irritant and can provoke skin lesions in the form of eczema and dermatitis."[2] Doesn't sound very healthy, does it?

If you still doubt the harm that may be caused by sodium lauryl sulfate and related substances, consider that these chemicals are powerful degreasers used to clean oil and other stains off the floor of auto repair shops. This shows how harsh these substances can be.

I advise using the mildest shampoos and conditioners you can find. Coconut-based products are a wonderful alternative to the harsh solutions that are so prevalent. If you're looking for a great way to make your hair silkier, consider jojoba oil. While taking an evening bath, work some jojoba oil into your wet hair and leave it in all night long. In the morning, wash the oil out. Your hair will be incredibly soft.

Hair Coloring Products

If you are intent on coloring your hair, please be careful and make sure you read the ingredients on the coloring product. Take the time to look for natural or "organic" coloring ingredients, or at least find those products with the fewest chemicals as possible, and especially avoid ammonia and alcohol. You may want to consider henna, an age-old herbal-based colorant that has worked well for centuries.

Hazards in the Hair Salon

Did you know that hair stylists are at high risk for health disorders? The increased incidence of disease is attributed to the frequent contact stylists have with beauty salon chemicals such as hair dyes. In fact, many beauticians eventually have to leave their profession due to the toxic nature of their work environment. According to an article published by the National Institute for Occupational Safety and Health, "Hairdressers should receive regular and repeated education about the potential hazards in the workplace."[3]

Lice Treatment Products

Every once in a while, schools report an outbreak of head lice among their pupils, and parents have to scramble for treatment products. If your child gets head lice, choose products that are pesticide- and chemical-free, and avoid dangerous substances such as the toxin piperonyl butoxide (PBU). Great alternatives include products that contain enzymes from natural vegetable extracts. These enzymes kill the head lice without the use of toxic chemicals that can be absorbed into your child's skin.

Encourage your child to avoid habits that can lead to head lice infestation. Head-to-head contact, which can occur when children bend over the same book, for instance; use of another child's comb, brush, hair accessory, or hat; and contact with another child's bedding can all lead to the spread of head lice. Warn your child against this type of contact, and he will be less likely to experience this common school-age problem.

Blow Dryers

Hair is composed of mostly protein, which can be damaged by high heat. Ideally, you should let your hair dry naturally, or perhaps towel-dry it before air-drying it, but who has the time? I suggest that you set your hair blow dryer on low heat to avoid the damage created by higher temperatures. This will help prevent overdrying and create fewer split ends.

Realize that some blow dryers use asbestos as insulation. Yes, little asbestos fibers have been known to fly out of these appliances. Because asbestos can be so harmful to lungs, it's important to buy asbestos-free blow dryers. (Refer to page 236 of the Resources section.)

SOAPS

When choosing a soap for the body or face, again think of products that contain coconut oil. As it cleans, this natural substance protects the skin by maintaining natural oils. Remember that you want your soaps to be gentle and moisturizing. There is no need to use harsh cleansers that will strip your skin of natural oils.

When you bathe your baby, use a very mild chemical-free soap. Most infants do not need a moisturizer unless they suffer from dry skin, in which case, the cause of the problem should be determined and addressed. Sometimes the dryness is caused by a lack of oil in the breast-feeding mother's diet, and sometimes, by a lack of oil in the infant's formula. Until the situation is corrected, apply a chemical-free moisturizer or a dab of coconut oil after your baby's bath.

Within the last few years, there has been a proliferation of antibacterial soaps on the market. Avoid these as much as possible. Yes, they will help kill the germs on your hands, but they can also get absorbed into your body, where they will eliminate the good bacteria as well as the bad. This will depress your natural defense system and foster the growth of harmful organisms, such as yeast. Scientists say that antibacterial soaps and cleansers—which, by the way, use antibiotics such as triclosan—will also help promote the growth of "super" antibiotic-resistant germs. If I have not yet convinced you that antibacterial soaps are not a good choice, consider that an article in the *Annals of Internal Medicine* concluded, "Evidence linking the use of antibacterial products to better health for the people who use them has been lacking."[4] Natural soap and water are a much better option.

OTHER SKIN-CARE PRODUCTS

When choosing face and body creams and lotions, I strongly suggest that you keep away from products that include polyethylene glycol or propylene glycol. These commonly used chemicals provide a slippery feel in lotions and creams, which is why they are so popular with manufacturers. Be aware, though, that these toxins are also used in antifreeze and brake fluid. Do you really want to apply them to your delicate skin?

As you age, skin loses its natural oils and becomes dry, leathery, and wrinkly. To combat this, you want to replenish the oils with substances that are as close as possible to the oils naturally present in skin. Both jojoba oil and coconut oil fit the bill. They are body-friendly and work well to maintain the skin's suppleness, softness, and smoothness. I use these oils straight out of the container, but you can also choose products that include these oils among other natural ingredients. Since jojoba oil is the less greasy of the two, I suggest applying this to your face during the day. It absorbs quickly and can even be used under makeup. Coconut oil is a bit heavier and makes a great night cream. It is also useful in healing skin that has been damaged by the harmful rays of the sun. (To learn more about this, see page 80 of Chapter 5.)

Another excellent skin-care product is royal jelly, a milky secretion of honey bees. Royal jelly contains an abundance of vitamins, minerals, amino acids, and gelatin, which is a form of collagen. I use this product as a light facial mask. Royal jelly helps maintain skin firmness and elasticity, and also aids the pores in detoxification. I sometimes even eat royal jelly! I would strongly suggest buying it at a health food store rather than trying to get it directly from a beehive, though!

Some people like to use a facial toner, but many toners contain some form of alcohol, which can be very drying. I have found that raw apple cider vinegar is great for cleansing and toning pores. Just spritz some on your face before applying your moisturizer. I like to dilute the vinegar with a little water because it makes it easier for the liquid to travel through the dispenser.

If you use shaving cream, look for all-natural products that contain herbs and essential oils. Avoid those that include a toxin called a-pinene, which can damage the immune system.

Should You Worry About Cosmetic Containers?

Most cosmetics—even those from health-conscious companies—do not come in containers made of the less-toxic plastics mentioned earlier in the book. Some companies recognize this and offer glass cosmetic containers into which you can transfer your products. Is this necessary? I believe it isn't. Although glass is the preferred choice, the plastic isn't being heated, so there is less chance of chemicals leaching into the product. I do, however, look for products that come in biodegradable containers that will eventually break down and be absorbed by the earth. This information is usually provided on the package label.

OILS AND CREAMS FOR PREGNANT AND NURSING MOTHERS

During pregnancy, many women get stretch marks as their tummies and breasts expand. A good preventative measure is applying coconut oil to the skin, as this will keep the skin soft and supple.

Many breast-feeding mothers use lanolin to help keep the areola and nipple from cracking and drying. Lanolin is obtained from sheep's wool, and if the sheep have been administered hormones and antibiotics, both the mother and baby can be exposed to these toxins. A good alternative is natural shea butter, which is obtained from the seeds of the African shea tree.

DEODORANTS AND ANTIPERSPIRANTS

Most adolescents and adults use either a deodorant or an antiperspirant. Unfortunately, deodorants often contain the antibacterial agent triclosan, and antiperspirants contain aluminum. As an alternative, consider aluminum-free baking soda to keep underarms dry and free of odor. Another good alternative is a natural deodorant crystal, which often contains a combination of natural mineral salts and aloe vera.

Toxic Shock Syndrome

Toxic shock syndrome (TSS) is a rare, life-threatening complication of bacterial infection. While the syndrome can affect anyone—man, woman, or child—it most commonly occurs in menstruating women who use tampons. The tampon encourages the growth of the bacteria *Staphylococcus aureus,* which is already in the vagina, by becoming a breeding ground for the germs.

Toxic shock usually starts out with a high fever and a rash that resembles a sunburn, and quickly becomes serious. Other symptoms may include a rapid drop in blood pressure, vomiting and diarrhea, severe muscle aches, headaches, disorientation, and seizures.

The risk for TSS increases when more absorbent synthetic tampons are used, so I advise you to use the least absorbent tampons that will keep you dry, and to choose a product that is chlorine-free and made of organic cotton. I also advise against young girls using tampons. Once a girl has matured into adulthood, her immune system is better able to fight the bacteria that cause this disorder. Until then, she should use chlorine-free, organic cotton pads. Under no circumstances do I recommend that women sleep while wearing tampons. If TSS symptoms do appear, get immediate medical attention so that appropriate treatment can begin.

Incredible Coconut Oil

In this chapter, I discuss how coconut oil makes a great moisturizer, as well as a beneficial ingredient in soaps. Actually, coconut oil is also an effective treatment for just about any skin problem, from diaper rash to fungal infections to psoriasis. It can also be applied to cuts and scrapes. Finally, when muscles or arthritic joints are sore, try blending a little coconut oil with jojoba oil and raw apple cider vinegar. Rub this therapeutic balm into the problem areas and enjoy not only pain relief, but also considerable moisturizing effects.

ORGANIC MAKEUP

Think about the number of hours makeup stays in contact with your skin after you apply it. Ten hours? Twelve hours? Since many ingredients that are on your skin can be absorbed into your body, it makes sense to avoid the numerous products that contain toxins. Many eye shadows contain a toxic chemical called iron oxide, and eyeliners contain ascorbyl palmitate, another toxin. A good number of lipstick formulas include the toxin paraffin, and blushers, foundations, concealers, mascara, and powders often contain parabens. According to the National Institute of Occupational Safety and Health, 884 chemicals used in cosmetics have been reported to the United States Government as toxic substances.[5] So much for government watchdogs!

Fortunately, many companies now produce organic makeup, including foundations, concealers, lipstick and gloss, blush, and more. These products contain natural ingredients, including truly healthful substances such as jojoba oil and other natural oils. I recommend looking for them in the health and beauty section of your local health food store. It may take time to find just the right products for your skin tone and type, but you will be rewarded with greater health and beauty down the road. In some large stores, you may even find a consultant who will help you put together a regimen that meets your needs.

Of course, if you follow the recommendations provided in this book regarding clean water and food, exercise, and more, it may not be long before you don't want to cover up your face. It has been my experience that as patients begin to radiate a natural beauty, they stop using makeup entirely or use only minimal products.

Cosmetic Exercises

As discussed on page 148, as you age, skin loses its natural oils and becomes drier. It also loses tone, as do the various muscles in your body. Although you can't stop the aging process, there are exercises you can do to maintain muscle tone. These exercises are quick and easy to perform, and I am confident you will be happy with the results. Remember the old adage, "Use it or lose it."

For the first facial exercise, place the tips of your fingers on top of your forehead and gently press your fingers down toward your eyebrows while raising your eyebrows up for a count of two. Repeat the exercise for ten repetitions.

For the next exercise place your thumb and index finger in the corners of each eye next to your nose and squint your eyes ten times, holding each squint for a couple of seconds.

Here's another exercise. Place your thumb and index finger on top of your upper cheek, and gently press your fingers downward toward your jaw as you raise your upper cheek muscles. Hold the position for a couple of seconds, and repeat the exercise for a total of ten reps.

Place one index finger on the tip of your nose. Flex the nose downward as if you were trying to bring the tip of the nose toward your lips. You should actually feel your finger moving downward. Hold each movement for a couple of seconds, and repeat the exercise for ten repetitions.

Here's a simple one. Draw your cheeks in, open your mouth wide, and while the mouth is open, make your lips go in and out like a fish. Hold each drawing-in for a couple seconds, and perform ten reps total.

For the last facial exercise, jut your lower jaw out in front of your upper jaw, and open and close your mouth a total of ten times.

Many people ask me what they can do to tone their neck muscles and lower jaw (jowl), as these areas show loss of firmness as we age. Simply perform the curl-ups described on page 61 of Chapter 4. Although designed for the stomach muscles, curl-ups tone the neck and jowl muscles as well.

The facial exercises described above may seem a bit silly—okay, very silly!—but really do help attain and maintain a natural toned look, with absolutely no expense or risk. The next time you see someone at a stoplight putting on her makeup, why not perform some of these simple facial exercises. Who knows, maybe you'll start a new trend!

SARA—A CASE STUDY

Sara, a college student, had first come to my clinic when her leg was injured at cheerleading practice. As I treated her injury, I noticed that she was wearing thick makeup. I asked how things were going at school, and she told me that school was stressful and that her skin had been breaking out lately. I empathized with her situation and then reviewed a game plan she could implement as a college student living in a dorm. One of my suggestions was to switch to natural, chemical-free makeup and facial hygiene products. It was my feeling that Sara's skin was reacting negatively to the irritating chemicals in her makeup and cleansers, and that if she changed to a natural coconut-based soap, raw apple cider vinegar toner, natural moisturizers (jojoba oil by day and coconut oil by night), and organic makeup, her complexion problems would be a thing of the past.

I didn't see Sara until her next semester break when she stopped by just to say hello. Sara told me how happy she was now that her face had cleared up. I asked her about the injury that I treated several months earlier, and she said, "What injury?" I guess that to a college girl, having a clear complexion seems a lot more important that healing a leg injury. Sara's parents were so pleased by their daughter's results that they, too, got on the road to health by incorporating the recommendations presented in this book, starting with clean water.

ORAL HYGIENE

When you consider that oral hygiene products are used *inside your mouth*, you realize how important it is to choose products that are toxin-free. For starters, I recommend using a toothpaste that contains no fluoride—a toxin I discuss in Chapter 1. (See page 13.) Instead, use aluminum-free baking soda or fluoride-free baking

Don't Forget Your Nails

Did you know that nail polish and nail polish remover can be very toxic to the body? Nail polish often contains a toxin called toluene, and most nail polish removers contain acetone. Both of these toxins can cause respiratory problems and skin irritation. Look for toxin-free, odorless nail polish and polish remover that is water- or herbal-based. Have you ever noticed that at a nail salon, technicians often wear masks over their nose and mouth? It's not because they don't want to be recognized; it's the toxic fumes from the polish and other products being used.

soda toothpaste. They will clean your teeth and give you fresh breath without any side effects. After brushing, I suggest swishing clean water around in your mouth, followed by spitting, to further cleanse your teeth. I personally use a Water Pik-type of instrument every evening, and it is quite effective.

Many people gargle with a commercial mouthwash every morning. It certainly gives your mouth a clean taste, but it probably also contains ethanol and perhaps even fluoride. I suggest using raw apple cider vinegar as a mouthwash. This versatile product will clean your mouth and give it a fresh taste and smell.

Most dentists recommend flossing, but many flosses are waxed and/or contain fluoride. Look for a fluoride-free unwaxed floss, which will discourage the formation of plaque without causing a waxy buildup between your teeth.

Finally, when you visit your dentist, request that he avoid using fluoride in your mouth. Many dentists are becoming more aware of the hazards of fluoride and employ alternative products. If you can, find a good holistic dentist in your area—someone who understands how common chemicals can affect the whole body, and makes it a practice to use healthy substitutes.

Contact Lens Solutions

If you wear contact lenses, look for solutions that are salt (saline) based and designed for people with sensitive eyes. These products are less likely to contain chemicals such as chlorohexidine and thimerosal (mercury), both of which are known toxins.

CONCLUSION

You want to look your best. But when you use man-made products to achieve this goal, you set yourself up for problems ranging from short-term rashes to serious health disorders that may take years to develop. Isn't it great to know that you can both look and feel great by using natural products that do their job without compromising your health? These products work along with your body, allowing it to detoxify, repair, and rebuild.

Congratulations. You have completed step fourteen on the road to beautiful health. And remember, Health is Wealth!

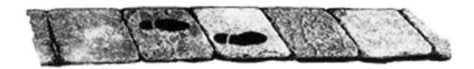

15. Clothing

What to wear.

Many people think that the clothing they wear has no impact on their health, other than its obvious use in keeping the body warm on a cold day or cool during hot weather. After all, clothes are worn on the *outside* of the body, so they can't affect the body's function, right? Well, no. Clothing that contains synthetic fibers or fibers grown and manufactured with chemicals can trigger a range of nasty physical reactions and, over time, can lead to a buildup of toxins within the body. Clothing that is too tight can interfere with body function and even cause infertility. And, as you know, inappropriate footwear can make it painful to carry out one of our most important activities—walking.

Fortunately, no matter your size or preferred style, you can find clothing and footwear that will keep you not only well dressed and comfortable, but also vibrantly healthy. This chapter explains how it's done.

CHOOSING THE BEST CLOTHING FIBERS

The best option when shopping for clothing is cotton products—preferably, "certified organic," which means that the fabrics were made without toxic chemicals. Although cotton was once considered the symbol of purity, it is now widely known that most cotton is grown in fields drenched in pesticides, and then processed with a blizzard of synthetic chemicals. Many of these chemicals are locked into fabrics and cannot be washed away in the laundry. When you wear clothes made of chemical-laden cotton—or any chemical-laden material, for that matter—the toxins can be absorbed through the skin and enter the bloodstream. While some are filtered through the liver and eliminated by the large intestine, many of these toxins are stored in tissue throughout the body. Over time, these substances can accumulate and cause a range of health problems.

It should be mentioned that pure cotton has important benefits as a clothing material. It wicks moisture from the skin and allows the skin to breathe, which

The Problem with Synthetic Fibers

In this chapter, you will learn that nylon, polyester, acrylics, and rayon expose your body to poisonous substances. Perhaps just as important, these fibers—unlike cotton and other natural materials—do not allow your body to breathe properly, and therefore hamper your skin's efforts to detoxify.

enables the skin to better eliminate toxins from the body and makes clothing comfortable for a longer period of time. Cotton also has a lower tendency to cause allergic reactions, which is especially important for infants, who have sensitive skin, and for anyone who has skin allergies. But cotton is not the only healthy material that you can wear. Silk, hemp, and wool are all natural fibers that can provide breathability, softness, and comfort. Just be sure to avoid wool if it causes you skin irritation, and choose organic fabrics whenever possible. Even non-organic cotton, silk, hemp, and wool are better options than synthetic fibers.

What types of fibers should be avoided? Nylon, polyester, acrylics, and rayon are created in vats of chemicals. This alone means that clothing made of these materials exposes your body to harmful toxins. During the garment-manufacturing process, further chemicals are used, many of which are known to contaminate the waste waters from textile manufacturing plants. Why would you want them contaminating your body as well?

AUBREY—A CASE STUDY

Aubrey was a very stylish patient. Whenever she came in for an appointment, she was well dressed. Many people complimented Aubrey on her taste in clothes, and this was important to her.

One day, Aubrey came to the clinic complaining that her upper back had been achy and itchy for about a week. I examined her back and discovered that there was nothing wrong with her spine and the surrounding musculature. The discomfort she was feeling seemed the result of a chemical reaction that had affected her skin. I asked her if she had been wearing any new clothes lately, and it was like asking a fish if it swims: Of course, she had been wearing new clothes. After checking the fabric labels, I suggested that she look for a more natural material (preferably cotton), and be sure to wear cotton underclothing. Aubrey went shopping for cotton underwear and outer garments that afternoon. The next day, she called to say that she was feeling much better and that her upper back pain and itch had disappeared.

HOSIERY AND UNDERGARMENTS

The undergarments you wear, including your hosiery, can have an enormous effect on your health simply because they are worn directly against your skin. There is no "buffer" between you and your underwear.

Nylon pantyhose creates the illusion of toned, tanned, flawless legs, free of varicose veins and other imperfections. This illusion comes at a price, though. The nylon does not allow your skin to breathe, permitting toxins to build up in your body. If you must wear pantyhose, I suggest that you slip into a bare-legged outfit when you get home. This will help open up the pores of your skin and allow for detoxification. Keep in mind, too, that if you follow the recommendations presented in this book regarding diet, exercise, and exposure to sunlight, you will not have to create the illusion of beautiful legs. You will actually have them because you will have addressed the cause of most problems.

When choosing women's panties, opt for all-cotton or silk items. Unlike nylon and other synthetic fabrics, cotton and silk are breathable and wick away the moisture that leads to vaginal infection. These fibers are also far less irritating to delicate skin.

The wearing of bras has been linked to an increased risk of breast cancer and other types of breast problems. A bra restricts the circulation of lymph, which normally carries away toxins and germs for elimination from the body. An article published in the *European Journal of Cancer* stated, "Premenopausal women who do not wear bras had half the risk of breast cancer compared with bra users."[1] Instead of a brassiere, you can simply wear a camisole or a well-fitted tank top under your clothes. This will give you some support, but won't restrict the circulation of lymph. If you don't feel comfortable going braless in the workplace and in public, at least remove your bra when you're at home and replace it with less restrictive clothing. Also avoid wearing a bra when you sleep so that you don't impede the functioning of your body all night long. In the morning, be sure to use the shower massage described on page 17 of Chapter 1. This will help keep the lymph flowing throughout your body so that it can remove harmful substances from your tissues.

No, I wasn't going to ignore the topic of men's underwear. For years, there has been a disagreement among men about whether to wear boxers or briefs. Briefs may look stylish and sexy to many men—and to many women, for that matter—but our Creator intended men's private parts to hang away from the body so that they remain cooler in temperature. When men wear briefs, the testicles are raised higher and closer to the body, causing a slight but detectable increase in the temperature of the testicles. This has been blamed for infertility in many men. The sperm are being "cooked"—not a pleasant thought, at least not for me. Men should therefore wear boxers for the health of their private parts and the maintenance of their fertility.

FOOT HEALTH AND FOOTWEAR

Healthy feet are the foundation of proper posture and, therefore, contribute to overall well-being. How can you keep your feet healthy? First, choose appropriate footwear that provides the protection your foot needs without creating constriction or imbalance. Then, whenever possible, take those shoes off so that you can build up important muscles through barefoot walking.

Choosing Footwear

When choosing footwear, as a first step, I suggest that you avoid sacrificing comfort for fashion. Just take a look at all the foot problems that we have in our society—corns, bunions, dropped arches, shortened ligaments and tendons, tight foot muscles, and weak foot muscles, not to mention far more serious problems. Your objective should be to avoid shoes that tend to cause these disorders.

I suggest that men and women alike wear "level" shoes, with just a slight heel, and choose a roomy toe box that does not cram toes together. As far as possible, avoid high heels, which, as most people know, put feet at an incredible biomechanical disadvantage. When high heels are worn, you are basically walking on your toes. An article printed in the *Journal of the American Podiatric Medical Association* stated, "One of the reasons that high heels may contribute to the contribution of hallux valgus [bunions] is that the wearers pronate during propulsion."[2] In other words, high heels place the individual's body weight on her toes, which causes a rolling in of the ankle (pronation). This stresses both the ankles and the feet. The constant wearing of heels can also shorten the Achilles tendon and calf muscles. Certainly, people were not meant to walk on their toes all the time. Even ballerinas take a break from toe shoes.

Wear High Heels Only When Necessary

Many more women are getting into the habit of wearing comfortable shoes or even sneakers to and from work. They carry their heels in their bags and slip into them when they arrive at the office. This minimizes heel-wearing time and gives feet a much needed rest. If possible, also kick off your heels while sitting down. Your boss may not appreciate your feet being propped up on the desk, so keep them hidden underneath and enjoy the sensation of gently stretching your toes.

What other guidelines should you keep in mind whenever you choose footwear? Look for shoes that leave your toes about one-half inch room between the end of the big toe and the end of the shoe, along with a broad-base heel of no more than one and one-half inches in height. Shoes should be made of natural components such as cotton and leather, and should be snug-fitting around the heel to prevent slippage. Avoid any seams and stitching that can rub your skin as you walk.

Building Foot Muscles

Earlier in the chapter, I mentioned that weak foot muscles are a major problem in our society. You see, shoes protect you from stubbing your toes and cutting your feet on abrasive surfaces, but worn over time, shoes also weaken the small muscles in your feet. Wearing shoes can be like wearing a cast on your feet. As a small boy, I suffered a broken arm and had to wear a cast for six weeks while the bone healed. When the cast was finally removed, I was shocked to see how my arm had shrunk (atrophied) from lack of use. This is what basically happens to your feet when they are always kept in shoes. Now, I realize a shoe is not as rigid as a cast, and therefore the muscles atrophy less than they would if your foot was totally immobilized, but some footwear can be a lot more rigid than other footwear, which can speed up the foot-weakening process. For example, work boots with steel toes and rigid arches, shoes that can't bend at the sole, and footwear made of reinforced fabrics tend to lock your foot into place. This type of footwear provides very important protection for people who do certain types of work, but over time, it can weaken the feet. Generally speaking, the less rigid your shoes are, the better off your feet will be.

If you compare your feet to those of a person who spends some time each day barefoot, you will see that their feet look more muscular. Try this experiment. While sitting in a chair with your bare feet on the floor, spread your toes as wide apart as you can and gently press your feet against the floor. You will see your foot muscles contracting as you spread your toes, and the muscles will be even more pronounced when you press your feet against the floor. Those little muscles that you've now seen in action give your feet the support they need to carry you around all day. When your feet are in shoes all the time, foot muscles become more relaxed because the muscles are supported and don't have to work as hard to propel the body forward. Over time, the muscles become weaker. The more rigid the shoe, the weaker the muscles become.

I have lost count of the many patients who appeared in my office with some sort of foot malady. After I treated their symptoms to make them more comfortable, I immediately looked for the cause of the problem. Most of the time, the root cause was a weakening of foot muscles. Even patients who walked all the time did so wearing shoes, which, as already explained, can be like mini-casts. When their immediate pain had been treated and relieved, I usually had them begin a regimen of barefoot walking. Initially, this meant kicking off their shoes as soon as they came home and spending a few minutes walking around on carpeting. Slowly, I had them increase their barefoot time until they kept their shoes off the entire evening. If they chose to spend some time outdoors, walking in the grass or in their garden, they were encouraged to do so. Soon, many of their foot and postural (spinal) aches and pains disappeared. I realize that some homes have hard surfaces that are unfriendly to bare feet. In my house, I keep soft slippers strategically placed at the opening of the bathroom and kitchen areas. This slipper idea may sound funny, but try it. Your feet will thank you. An article published in the *New Zealand Medical Journal* postulated that "Barefoot walking represents the best condition for the development of a healthy foot."[3] Strong feet equal healthy feet.

In Chapter 5, I discussed how you can benefit from placing your bare feet on the grass with the sun gently shining on your body to create a powerful recharging of the body through the energy emanating from the Earth and sun. This is a way to help not only your feet, but your whole body. I do suggest, however, that you stay away from sidewalks and other hard surfaces while your feet are bare.

Using Orthotics

Orthotics are shoe inserts designed to support the foot and/or relieve pain. While orthotics are helpful to some people, if they are being prescribed only for support, I suggest that you consider building up your foot muscles through barefoot walking. This can give your feet internal strength, making orthotics unnecessary. If you do choose to wear orthotics to relieve pain in the immediate future, ask your doctor how long you will have to wear the supportive devices and if and when you can be weaned from them. Just keep in mind that every foot problem is different, and that in your case, you may actually require orthotics whenever you wear shoes. Discuss this with your healthcare practitioner.

If just one foot requires treatment with a shoe insert, request that you also receive an insert for the other foot so that it will keep you level when you walk. Most people require two orthotic devices. But again, remember that each situation is different. In some cases—for instance, when one leg is shorter than the other—it may actually be necessary to use only one orthotic device.

ROBIN—A CASE STUDY

Robin came to my clinic complaining of foot discomfort. Her right forefoot was a bit swollen and actually felt hot to the touch. I could see the pain she was experiencing when I asked her to stand up and take a few steps in my examining room. I examined her feet, and they were like an infant's feet—very soft and very weak, with little to no muscular support. The ligaments were shortened, her arches had collapsed, and the bones in the front of her foot seemed crammed together. I looked at her footwear. No wonder she was in pain! The high-heeled stilts she was jamming her feet into were causing all kinds of biomechanical problems. I advised her to lay off the high heels for a month or so while I treated her. Then she could start barefoot walking in her home to strengthen her muscles. "No way!" Robin exclaimed. She would not give up her high heels—not even for a few weeks. She would not switch to flat shoes with a wider toe box.

Six months later, I was giving a healthcare seminar when I saw a hand go up in the back of the room. It was Robin. After hobbling up to the front of the room on her crutches, she proceeded to take off her high-top tennis shoe and display the surgical scar that ran along the top of her foot. With tears in her eyes, Robin said that the surgery might have been unnecessary if she had listened to my earlier advice.

Finally, Robin was ready to begin the road to health. I modified her program to accommodate her temporary inability to walk. She incorporated swimming and deep-water jogging in her day, she started to drink clean water and eat clean food, and she followed the other recommendations presented throughout the chapters in this book. She even prepared her food in glass cookware, used toxin-free cosmetics, and wore organic clothing. Robin's foot healed and she was able to walk without pain. Just as important, her lifestyle changes allowed her to experience a sense of overall health and well-being.

Considerations for Joggers and Runners

There are a lot of high-priced running and walking shoes on the market these days. Many shoe companies claim that you need the latest whiz-bang shoe with extra cushioning so you will experience less running-related injuries. When I walk or run, I try to stick with the simplest running shoe I can find. I choose a shoe that doesn't have extra padding and that doesn't flare out at the heels, as this causes unnecessary pronation (rolling or rotation) of the ankles and knees, causing stress to the legs and spine. I realize that some runners and walkers may find the "air clouds" to be just what they need. Certainly, people with special foot or joint problems may require shoes with extra padding. But for the majority of us, the less expensive, simpler shoes are probably healthier than the expensive high-tech models.

Many runners are now spending more time training barefoot on tracks and soft surfaces to help strengthen their feet. The runners with the strongest feet are generally those with the fewest foot and leg injuries. When you run barefoot, your feet have a natural tendency to land more on the arches of your feet, and then spring off the toes. Shoes hamper this action. The fact is that in other parts of the world, many of the greatest runners train by running barefoot for miles.

If you want to begin barefoot running, start a routine of walking barefoot on a soft surface, such as a grassy park or rubberized running track, for at least thirty minutes a session, three times a week, for six weeks. Dirt trails are fine, but be very careful to avoid debris such as rocks and sticks, which can puncture your skin. Definitely stay off sidewalks and asphalt. When you begin running, for the first week, cut down your walking session by five minutes, and spend just five minutes running without shoes. Each week, walk for five fewer minutes and add that time to your running routine. In six weeks, you'll be running barefoot for an entire thirty-minute workout. If you want to run longer than this, I suggest that you put on your running shoes for the remainder of the session.

CONCLUSION

What you wear is not just a matter of style, but also a matter of health. By choosing clothes made of natural fibers—ideally, organic—you will allow your body to function as it should and avoid filling it with toxic chemicals. To preserve or improve the health of your feet, avoid high heels as much as possible, and spend some time walking barefoot in order to strengthen your foot muscles. By following these simple guidelines, you will be far more likely to have a healthy body, mind, emotional and social well-being, and soul, as well. You have completed step fifteen on your journey down the road to magnificent health.

Remember, Health is Wealth!

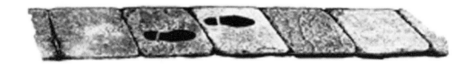

16. Household Cleaners and the Home Environment

I don't do windows.

If you're like most people, you probably don't enjoy cleaning your house but think of it as a necessary inconvenience—something that you have to do so that your home looks good and is free of dust, dirt, and germs. Because you want to get every surface clean with the least amount of fuss, you may be intrigued by the endless stream of cleaning products advertised on television. After all, who doesn't want sparkling results in record time? There's just one problem: Many of these products contain toxic chemicals that pose dangers to your health, as well as the health of your family and your pets.

Is there a way to get your house clean without all those toxins? Absolutely. This chapter begins by talking about the dangers posed by many common cleansers and recommends alternatives that can help you safely clean every area of your house as well as your laundry, dishes, and more. The chapter then suggests simple changes that you can make in your home—such as substituting a hemp shower curtain for a plastic curtain—that will create a healthier home environment and, in some cases, even shorten the dreaded task of cleaning.

CHEMICAL TOXINS IN THE HOME

The American Lung Association warns, "Household cleaning agents, personal care products, pesticides, paints, hobby products, and solvents may be a source of hundreds of potentially harmful chemicals."[1] When you think about it, that statement is pretty staggering because it means that we are introducing dozens and dozens of poisons into our own homes, often through products that we believe are going to make our environment cleaner, safer, and just plain *better*. Because these products are usually inhaled during and after use—as they linger on floors, countertops, and other surfaces—they can do real harm to the respiratory and central nervous systems, and can also cause or aggravate allergies. If they are handled without gloves, they come into contact with the skin and can be absorbed into the body much like the cosmetics discussed in Chapter 14. In fact, household toxins found in cleansers and other household products have been linked to a wide range of problems affecting all body systems. Generally, the more contact you have with chemicals over time, the greater the risk of experiencing long-term health problems. Keep in mind, too, that when toxin-containing laundry detergents, dishwashing liquids, etc., are discharged into municipal waste water, they pollute the environment.

As you have already gathered, the list of toxic chemicals that may be found in household cleaners is long—too long to include in this book. Some of the most common substances are acetone, alcohol, ammonia, benzene, chlorine bleach, fluorocarbons, formaldehyde, phosphates, and sodium hydroxide. In what products can these be found? Again, the potential list is extensive, and includes air fresheners, all-purpose cleaners, bathroom cleaners, dishwashing liquids, laundry detergents, fabric softeners, dusting sprays, stove and oven cleaners, floor-cleaning products, carpet-cleaning products, and more.

It is hard to be familiar with every toxic substance that may be used in commercial cleaning products, so you may want to use a few rules of thumb. First, if it smells strong, it probably is toxic. If the label warns you to use in only in a well-ventilated room, or the product makes your eyes tear or your throat feel raw, it's probably *very* toxic. If the names of the ingredients are too long to pronounce and sound like they came out of a test tube, they probably did, and you don't want them in your home.

CHOOSING NATURAL CLEANERS

Despite the large number of toxin-laden cleaning products found in every supermarket, these days, there are also plenty of safe and effective options for the health-conscious individual. You can, of course, opt for simple, natural cleaning substances like white vinegar, which has been used for decades. Or you can take advantage of the wealth of natural cleaning products that are now available not only in health food stores, but also in your average supermarket. Look for products that contain natural ingredients such as aloe vera gel, citric acid, corn- and coconut-derived surfactants, proteolytic enzymes, plant oils, and the like. You can even find non-chlorine bleach. Products are available for different needs, from cleaning the kitchen floor to doing the laundry. In some cases, cleansers include a natural fragrance so that your kitchen or bath will smell like a fresh cucumber or a field of lavender after it has been cleaned. If you prefer unscented products, those are available, too. (Look for words like "free and clear," which also indicate the absence of dyes.) These cleaners are good not only for your family, but also for the environment as the ingredients are biodegradable.

Why Are Enzymes in My Laundry and Dish Detergents?

Enzymes are used in cleaning and fabric-care products because of their ability to break down larger water-insoluble stains into smaller more water-soluble pieces. The smaller pieces are then removed from the clothing or dishes through the mechanical use of water and/or interaction with other detergent ingredients. A small quantity of these natural enzymes can replace a large amount of man-made cleaning agents. Enzymes also work well at low temperatures and are completely biodegradable.

BATHROOM CARE

The bathroom is one of the areas of the home where people are especially likely to use harsh, potentially hazardous cleaning products. After all, you want your bathroom to look clean and smell fresh, and you should remove any mildew or soap scum that has formed on tiles and glass. It seems like an occasion to take out the "big guns."

As already discussed in this chapter, there are many new all-natural products that are designed to clean the different surfaces found in the bathroom. I also recommend good old-fashioned baking soda. Widely available, this substance makes a great scouring powder and works as an all-purpose cleaner, as well. Use this product to clean your toilet bowl, tile walls and floors, and sink. When finished cleaning, simply wipe up the powder or wash it down the drain.

If you have mold and mildew problems in your bathroom, look specifically for a product with natural vegetable-derived surfactants. These will eliminate the unwanted mold without resorting to the ammonia and chlorine found in common tub and tile cleaners. Products made with lavender oil or another natural oil will leave your bathroom smelling clean and fresh, which is much better than the tear-producing toxic fumes of standard tile cleaners.

While we're considering the bathroom, let's look at some simple changes you can make that will leave your bathroom a little safer and easier to clean. If you find mold growing on your shower curtain, use hemp as an inside liner. Mold has a really tough time growing on hemp.

To discourage mold from growing elsewhere in your bathroom, wipe down your shower tiles with a bath towel after your shower, and then hang up the bath towel so it can dry. If you have a bathroom exhaust fan, run it during your shower and for thirty minutes or so afterwards to help eliminate the moisture. If necessary, hook up a timer to the fan so that it will shut itself off after the desired period of time. If you don't have an exhaust fan and weather permits, open the bathroom window for a half hour or so. If mold and mildew are a persistent problem in your house, consider having a thermidistat hooked up to your heating and cooling system. This will allow you to control both temperature *and* humidity.

The next time you're in your local hardware store, look for nontoxic water-based sealants and caulking that can be applied around your bathtub and elsewhere to prevent mold growth. Silicone is a nontoxic caulking base. Avoid products that contain formaldehyde, butyl rubber, neoprene, and acrylic, all of which will *off-gas*—release toxic gaseous chemicals—into your home.

KITCHEN CARE

Like your bathrooms, your kitchen is fairly high maintenance, and the more you use it, the more care it requires.

If your kitchen is partly tiled, many of the same cleaners used in your bathroom will work on your kitchen's tiled floors, walls, backsplashes, and counters. In kitchens, you are usually less concerned with soap scum and mildew and more challenged by grease and food particles that can splatter during cooking. Again, look for natural all-purpose cleaners and dishwashing liquids. When buying dishwashing liquids, vegetable-based surfactants make an excellent choice. Products that contain orange and lemon extracts are especially effective.

You don't have to be a chemist to realize that oven cleaners are full of hazardous chemicals. Even if you couldn't smell those toxins a mile away, all the warnings printed on the product label would alert you to the fact that this is not a safe product to use around family members or pets. As a nontoxic but highly effective alternative, I recommend baking soda. Sprinkle baking soda over the oven bottom until the powder is about one-quarter inch thick. Then use a spray bottle to spray the baking soda with water just until the product is damp. Now walk away—really! No rubbing is necessary. Whenever you think of it, spray the baking soda with water to rewet it. The next day, you will be able to effortlessly remove the baking soda—and all the baked-on grime—with a wet sponge. Rinse out the white residue and your oven will be ready for action again. Just as important, you'll know that your next meal won't absorb chemicals from your oven.

Keep in mind that baking soda will clean, scour, and deodorize just about any surface—not just ovens. Use it on counters and sinks, pour it down the kitchen drain to make it sweet-smelling, and use it to wipe down the inside of refrigerators. Don't forget to keep an open box in the fridge to help deodorize between cleanings.

Want another simple, easy-to-find, inexpensive kitchen cleaner? Combine distilled white vinegar with water, using a fifty-fifty mix. I suggest keeping the solution in a spray bottle so that you can squirt it on any area that needs attention.

DUSTING AND VACUUMING

Once your bathroom and kitchen have been washed, you'll have completed the lion's share of cleaning in your house. But you'll still want to remove dust and dirt from the furniture and floors in other rooms of the house.

Instead of using a toxin-laden product designed to attract dust to the cloth, simply dampen a soft lint-free cloth a bit with water. This will help ensure that the dust ends up on the cloth and isn't simply moved to another part of the surface. If you want to add a protective layer of oil to your wood furniture, skip commercial furniture polishes, which contain naptha, diglycol laurate, and other chemicals that are central nervous system depressants and neurotoxins. Instead look for a natural product whose main ingredients are water and olive or orange oil.

Even if you don't have allergies, I recommend using a vacuum cleaner whose filtration system removes both dirt and allergens as you clean. A HEPA filter (high efficiency particulate air filter) can be especially effective at picking up pollen, dust, and other particles. Vacuum at least once week, especially over carpeted areas. Also make sure to change the vacuum cleaner bag on a regular basis and in a well-ventilated area. This will help keep the machine's suction at an optimum level and prevent you from inhaling dust and dirt. Do not choose a bagless vacuum cleaner, as it is far less sanitary than a machine that includes a bag. Consider this: Would you dump trash into your kitchen garbage can without using a liner that could be removed?

If you are having a home built or renovated, consider installing a central vacuum system. With this system, a central power unit is mounted in an out-of-the-way place such as the basement or garage. Inlet valves are then positioned throughout the house and connected to the central power unit through ducts. You simply plug the vacuum hose in an inlet and begin vacuuming; the system carries the dirt from the room through the power unit, where it is deposited in a canister or bag. Since the bag has to be disposed of only every six months or so, you have less contact with dirt and debris.

PRODUCTS FOR THE LAUNDRY ROOM

As you know by now, most commercial cleaners, including laundry products, contain toxins. Substances such as petroleum-derived surfactants, benzyl acetate, phosphates, synthetic fragrances, and chlorine bleach can be breathed in or absorbed through the skin, and cause a host of health problems. And these products are just as bad for the environment as they are for you.

Instead of using standard contaminant-laden laundry detergents, look for products that contain nontoxic, biodegradable, plant-derived ingredients such as corn, palm kernel, and coconut oil. Enzymes are another good ingredient. As mentioned on page 165, these natural substances can break up food stains both naturally and effectively, reducing the amount of detergent needed.

When stains are tough, instead of using a conventional stain remover, try white distilled vinegar. Just saturate the stain with the vinegar, allow it to sit for a few minutes, and rinse with cool water. Repeat the process until the stain is gone, and launder the garment as usual. White distilled vinegar also makes a wonderful nontoxic fabric softener. Just add one-eighth cup to your laundry load.

The Healthier Dry Cleaning Option

While some clothing labels say "Dry Clean Only," and many people have even washable garments dry cleaned for the sake of convenience, conventional dry cleaning routinely uses toxic chemicals such as perc (perchloroethylene), which can easily be absorbed into your body. How much can perc affect your health? An article published in the *American Journal of Industrial Medicine* concluded, "Wives of dry cleaners were more than twice as likely to have a history of attempting to become pregnant for more than 12 months or to have sought care for an infertility problem."[2] In other words, constant exposure to perc can actually decrease fertility.

Instead of having your clothes dry cleaned, consider the possibility of hand-washing these items at home. If this is either inadvisable or unfeasible, be aware of the option of professional wet cleaning. When you have your clothes wet cleaned, they are washed in computer-controlled washers and dryers that gently clean the clothes, sometimes spinning as slowly as six revolutions per minute. Water-based stains—which make up the majority of stains—generally come out quickly. Any remaining stains are removed using specialized water-based pre-spotting solutions. Since just about every dry cleanable garment can be wet cleaned with the use of far fewer chemicals, wet cleaning represents a healthier option for consumers who want their clothes to be as safe as they are clean.

Although washing clothes in cold water uses less energy, there is one time that I suggest using hot water—when washing underwear. These garments not only get sweaty, but can get contaminated with fecal matter. For this reason, I urge you to wash your undergarments with hot water and dry them on high heat.

As long as we're on the subject of drying clothes, I'd like to mention that hanging your clothes on an outside line is still the healthiest and most energy-efficient way to go. But if (like most people), you opt to use a dryer, I do suggest that you clean your lint filter regularly—preferably, after each load of laundry is complete. This will allow for more efficient heat flow and will also prevent fires that can occur when the heat of the dryer ignites a buildup of lint. Be aware, too, that the electrical components of your dryer contain PBDE (polybrominated diphenyl ether), a flame-retardant chemical that is toxic. This chemical can contaminate dryer lint, so when you clean your lint filter, dispose of the lint as quickly as possible without breathing it in.

AIR FRESHENERS AND DEODORIZERS

Many people use commercial air fresheners in bathrooms and other parts of their home to cover up unwelcome odors and add a pleasant scent to the room. But while air fresheners may smell nice, they contain harmful chemicals, including benzyl acetate, which can be irritating to the eyes, mucous membranes, and respiratory tract.

Fortunately, essential oils provide a safe way to add scent to your home. Extracted from plants such as lavender and rosemary, these oils are potent, but contain no chemicals that can turn home sweet home into an environmental hazard. There are many ways of dispersing these oils, too. For instance, you can simply place a few drops of lavender essential oil on a napkin and position the napkin in the corner of a room, where it will release its scent into the air. (This works in cars, too.) If you're willing to spend a little more money, you can buy an essential-oil diffuser, which is a mini-vaporizer that gently emits a fragrant mist throughout the house. Another option is a reed diffuser. Reeds sit in a bottle of essential oil, absorb the oil, and disperse it throughout the room. Any of these methods will scent your house safely, without toxic chemicals and without posing a fire hazard, as candles do. If you do choose to use candles, though, buy toxin-free candles made of beeswax or soy.

Before we leave the subject of air fresheners, please be aware that the air fresheners you buy for the car are just as toxic as those created for the home. Again, if you find that the odor in your car is objectionable, use the essential oil of your choice to scent your car.

AIR FILTERS AND PURIFIERS

Earlier, we discussed how you can safely add pleasant scents to the rooms of your home. However, a more important subject is air quality.

Most forced-air home heating and air conditioning units have filters that need to be changed at regular intervals of a month to several months. Have you ever taken a good look at your filters? If you hold them up to the light, you can actually see through most of them. Because many are so cheaply made, they often do not do a good job of trapping pollens and other dust particles that float in the air. Moreover, many are made of fiberglass, which means that dangerous fiberglass particles can become dislodged and drift into the air, where you can breathe them in.

Instead of using cheaply made throw-away filters, I suggest having filters custom-made for your larger air returns. These custom filters are much heavier and denser than disposable filters. Many are made of horsehair, and some are composed of heavy mesh. About once a month, wash out the filter, air dry it for about an hour (while your unit is off), and then reinstall it. The denser filters trap a great deal more airborne pollen, mold, dust, and other pollutants, making your home environment cleaner and purer. Make sure, however, that the filter does not restrict airflow; otherwise, you will stress your heating and cooling unit. You should be able to feel air flow by placing your hand up to your return vent.

If you do not have access to custom-made air filters or you simply don't want to wash them every month, look for store-bought pleated nonfiberglass filters. Pleated filters are efficient at trapping airborne particles because of the larger surface area created by the pleats. Buy one that has a MERV (minimum efficiency reporting value) rating of at least eleven. All filters come with an industry standard rating that ranges from one to twelve. A filter with a rating of eleven will trap 85 to 90 percent of the airborne particles in your home. These filters come in a one-inch thickness that is compatible with most forced-air systems. They can be used for three months before they have to be replaced.

If you are concerned about microorganisms and other potentially harmful airborne particles, consider having a point-of-entry ultraviolet bulb attached either directly to your heating and cooling unit, or inside the duct next to the unit. As the air circulates through the house, it passes in front of an ultraviolet bulb that emits a very low ozone discharge. This kills mold spores, viruses, bacteria, and other harmful particles. After the bulb renders the particles harmless, the filter traps them. This device can be easily installed by most heating and cooling companies, and the bulbs generally need to be replaced only every year or two as they burn out.

Although I prefer the point-of-entry air purification system discussed above, many people like free-standing floor air purifiers that treat a smaller area of the home, such as a bedroom or office. If you opt for this type of purifier, look

Solar Panels

If you're interested in going greener and tapping into free heat from the sun, consider installing solar panels on your roof. Although solar panels will probably not meet all your heating needs, they can usually produce enough energy to heat the water in your home or your swimming pool.

for one with a HEPA filter, and be sure to change the filter as often as directed by the manufacturer—usually, about twice a year.

No matter what the temperature is outside, and even if you have an air purification system in your home, it's a good idea to allow some fresh air to get into your house. As first discussed on page 101 of Chapter 7, I suggest that you leave one window cracked open about a quarter of an inch at all times. Another natural way to freshen up a home is to hang plants throughout the house. Plants convert carbon dioxide into oxygen, which, as you know, is a natural dextoxifier.

BETHANY—A CASE STUDY

Bethany was brought into my clinic by her husband, Jim. The previous evening, Jim had arrived home to find that Bethany was not feeling well. When Bethany visited my clinic, she was still suffering from a wide range of symptoms, including numbness of her hands, tingling in her feet, a variety of aches and pains, fatigue, and depression. Just twenty-four hours earlier, Bethany had been feeling fine, and she didn't know why she was suddenly so ill.

During my examination, I asked Bethany and Jim about their home environment and especially about their furnace. Jim reported that their furnace had been "acting funny"—shutting down and restarting, and making weird noises. I realized that Bethany was probably suffering from carbon monoxide poisoning. After treating Bethany for her aches and pains, I immediately put her on a twenty-four hour detoxification lemon water fast. Most important, I instructed Jim to have the furnace fixed and to stay out of the house until it was in good working order. It was a nice day outside, so I advised Bethany to remain out-of-doors most of the day and to breathe deeply to help flush the carbon monoxide out of her system. I also instructed the couple to have the heating people air out the house after the furnace was fixed. Jim would install a plug-in carbon monoxide detector so that further problems like this simply would not happen, and he would also add a point-of-entry ultraviolet bulb along with an upgraded air filter to their home.

In a couple of days, Bethany was feeling like her old self again, and she and Jim were enjoying a cleaner, purer home environment.

INSECT AND PEST CONTROL

Routine and thorough house cleaning can help prevent bug infestations by removing the food particles that attract insects and by disturbing or vacuuming away insects and their eggs. But even the cleanest home can be invaded by ants and other pests.

As much as possible, avoid using commercial pesticides in and around your house. Most pesticides contain highly toxic chemicals such as mancozeb and chlorophthalic anhydride, which pose danger to you, your children, and your pets. At the very least, these chemicals can cause eyes to tear and aggravate allergies. In the worst case scenarios, pesticides can cause serious illness.

White distilled vinegar poured around the foundation of the house is a wonderful way to keep ants from entering your home. Peppermint soap or oil is another great insect repellent that can be used safely around your home's perimeter and even indoors. Simply mix up some peppermint soap or a few drops of oil with water in a spray bottle, and spray along the baseboards or foundation of your home. This mixture can also help keep rodents such as mice away. When large pests such as bats and raccoons become a nuisance, try using an ultrasonic device that creates an electronic "fence" by emitting sounds that are disturbing to animals but cannot be heard by humans.

If you must use a pesticide in your home, be sure to get your family—including your pets—out of the house for a few days and keep a window open to air out the home. If chemicals must be used around your home's perimeter, make sure that pets and children do not come in contact with them. If necessary, have your kids play in a park for a couple of weeks—not on your lawn or around your house.

If you and your family need protection from insects when spending time outdoors, avoid using toxic bug repellents, such as commercial products that contain DEET (N,N-diethyl-meta-toluamide). Instead, opt for natural bug repellents, such as those containing essential oils. A couple of drops of lemon or peppermint oil rubbed into the skin make an effective mosquito repellent.

HOME RENOVATION AND REDECORATING

Periodically, most homeowners redecorate one or more rooms, and occasionally, they make more substantial renovations. While this is a great way to make your home look more attractive, you should be aware that this is also a time when you'll be adding new materials in the form of paint and other wall coverings, flooring, and maybe even countertops, cabinets, and furniture. Depending on what you choose, this can make your home environment more or less healthy for your family. That's why it's so important to make educated choices whether you're simply repainting a room or doing major reconstruction.

The Kitchen

If you are thinking of renovating your kitchen, explore materials that are free of toxins and unlikely to off-gas toxic chemicals into your environment. Although hardwood and tile floors can contain the toxin formaldehyde, they don't off-gas to the extent that carpeting does. True linoleum—which is getting hard to find—is a safe choice because it is made of linseed oil and other natural materials. Be aware that PVC flooring is sometimes *referred* to as linoleum, but is a very different material, and will off-gas. Consider this when planning your renovation.

Some countertops, such as Formica, will off-gas formaldehyde. Corian is a safer choice. Although granite countertops seem like a natural and healthy option, they have been found to emit radon, a cancer-causing odorless natural gas. If you currently have granite countertops, you can have your kitchen (and the rest of your home) checked for radon emissions. For these and other household materials—including flooring—nontoxic water-based sealants may be the most cost-effective answer. You apply the sealant one time only, and it locks the chemicals into the material to prevent off-gassing.

Finally, if you are planning to install new kitchen cabinets, consider solid oak, cherry, maple, or hickory, as these materials will not off-gas chemicals. Cabinets made of plywood or particle board can emit toxins, especially formaldehyde, and should be sealed.

Carpeting

Carpeted floors are very comfortable and make it much more pleasant to walk around the house in bare feet, as I suggest in Chapter 15. The main drawback is that the carpets themselves and the materials used to lay them can off-gas toxins such as formaldehyde and 4-PC (4-phenylcyclohexene) for up to five years after the carpet has been installed. So if you're thinking of laying down new carpet in your home, there are some things you should keep in mind.

An article published in *The Environmental Magazine* reported, "When the Environmental Protection Agency came down with sick building syndrome in its Washington DC headquarters back in 1998, the irony was lost on no one. Health problems there erupted after installation of new carpeting. Suspicion hovered around chemical by-product emissions from carpet backing and adhesives."[3] The carpet was replaced and the health problems disappeared.

If you love the look and feel of carpeting but don't want the chemicals, first try to purchase nontoxic carpets and area rugs made of wool, sisal, or another natural material. Wool padding is also available.

If you are moving into a new home and are using commercial-grade carpeting that was manufactured with chemicals, have it installed at least a week before you move in. This will give the carpeting, the padding, and other materials time to off-gas as much as possible. If you are having new carpeting installed in your existing home, open the windows and use fans to move the toxins out of your house. Another option is to unroll the carpeting and allow it to off-gas in a garage or other protected area for a week or so before you have it laid. That way, it will do much of its off-gassing before it enters your living area.

When the new carpet is finally in place, deep-clean it with water and vinegar or with a natural carpet shampoo that contains vegetable surfactants. Follow this with a natural water-based carpet sealer to prevent further off-gassing.

Painting and Wallpaper

Believe it or not, paints are a major source of indoor air pollution. The EPA (Environmental Protection Agency) lists paint among the top five environmental hazards. The chief danger posed by paint is its volatile organic compounds, or VOCs, which include formaldehyde, benzene, toluene, and other chemicals. Emissions from these VOCs can continue up to a year after paint is applied.

When you paint your home, look for a product that lists the level of VOCs as 50g/L (50 grams per liter) or less. You can even purchase paints and primers with a VOC level of 0g/L, which means that no toxic off-gassing will occur. More and more paint companies are offering these safer products as consumers become increasingly aware of indoor pollution. If you use a paint that has a high level of VOCs, look for a water-based product and wear a respirator mask when applying the paint. Then keep the windows open and the air moving until that new-paint smell is gone.

Be aware that paint manufactured before 1978 may contain lead, and paint manufactured before 1950 can be 50-percent lead. If you have an older home and older paint, you'll want to cover it up with a newer, less toxic product. If lead paint is peeling off your walls or other surfaces, hire a professional with experience in lead paint removal to eliminate the paint safely.

If you decide to wallpaper your rooms instead of painting them, choose your wallpaper carefully, as there can be a big difference between products. Some wallpaper is made of polyvinyl chloride (PVC), which can off-gas toxins into the room. Instead, choose wallpaper that is made of a natural cloth fiber such as organic cotton, or look for a paper product that is certified FSC (Forest Stewardship Council). You also want your wallpaper to include water-based inks and adhesives.

Asbestos Insulation and the Older Home

Many older homes have asbestos insulation wrapped around the pipes. If this is true of your home, don't try to remove the insulation yourself because this process releases dangerous filaments into the air. Instead, hire a company that specializes in asbestos removal.

Window Coverings

Many window coverings—including blinds, shades, and curtains—contain the toxin formaldehyde. As an alternative, look for coverings made of cotton, bamboo, or hemp. Natural wood is also a nice choice. If you are in doubt about the chemicals used in the manufacture of these items, try to close off the room from the rest of the house and leave the windows open for about a week after the coverings are installed. This will give the chemicals time to off-gas.

Protecting Ductwork

If you are having major construction done on your home—or if you are having a new home built—ask the builder to place plastic covers over the air ducts during the construction process. Most builders will be happy to do this for you and it's an important precaution, as you don't want to turn on your heat or air conditioning and have dust blow into your home. You may even want to have an air duct vacuuming company vacuum out the ductwork once construction has been completed. This is a great way to help insure that your home is as clean as it is beautiful.

Adding New Insulation

Insulation is a great means of helping your house stay warm in the winter and cool in the summer without using more fossil fuel. Many types of insulation contain fiberglass. While an effective form of insulation, fiberglass poses a health hazard when fibers become loose and float into the air. If you have fiberglass insulation and it is coming loose, speak to specially trained professionals about sealing or removing the material. If you are adding new insulation, look into natural products. Both cotton and wool insulation are safe alternatives, and wool is naturally flame-retardant.

Adding New Upholstered Furniture

New upholstered couches and chairs often contain foam that can off-gas toxic PBBs, or polybrominated biphenyls, a chemical that's added to the padding to help prevent it from catching on fire. The furniture may also contain flame-retardant chemicals such as hexabromocyclododecane, and the fabric may be treated with stain-resistant substances such as Teflon.

If possible, choose furniture that has been made with nontoxic foam or cotton padding. Look for fabrics like wax-coated cotton for stain protection, and select wool barrier materials that naturally prevent the spread of flames. These choices will help ensure that your new acquisitions are not only practical, but also safe for you and your family.

CONNIE—A CASE STUDY

Connie came into my clinic complaining of body aches and nausea. When I examined Connie, I found nothing that would cause her to have these symptoms. But as we spoke, the source of her illness became clear.

A week earlier, Connie and her husband had moved into a new home, which they had built together. Connie couldn't stop talking about her new kitchen cabinets and new furnishings. I explained to her that all of the beautiful things in her dream house were causing her to be sick through the off-gassing of chemicals. Connie didn't have to move, but the house needed time to rid itself of the more volatile substances found in new paint, carpeting, window shades, etc. This would be a perfect time for Connie and her husband to enjoy a get-away while professionals aired out their house and used natural sealants on carpets, tiles, hardwood floors, cabinets, decks, and the garage floor. A twenty-four-hour water and lemon juice fast would help rid her body of the chemicals she had already absorbed, solving Connie's immediate problems. Further, I suggested that when Connie returned home, she clean the rooms using only nontoxic products and implement the other lifestyle components discussed in this book.

When Connie and her husband came back from their trip, their house was free of the airborne chemicals that had been making Connie so ill. As the couple changed their diet, introduced better sleeping habits, and made other positive changes, their sense of well-being was further enhanced. To this day, Connie is happy and healthy in her dream home.

THE BABY'S ROOM

An infant doesn't have the detoxifying capabilities of an older individual. That's why you have to be especially careful when creating a room for your baby.

I know of many parents who, as soon as they learn that a baby is on the way, start to redecorate the infant's room with new carpet, new paint, and new curtains. Unfortunately, these very well-meaning parents are loading the room up with airborne toxins that will stress the infant's body.

It's best to prepare your child's room as much in advance of his birth as possible so that the new materials have time to somewhat off-gas prior to his arrival. Another option is to use sealants to prevent off-gassing. Just as important, follow the suggestions presented earlier in this chapter when choosing paint, carpeting, etc. Low VOC paint, natural flooring, cotton curtains, and other non- or low-toxin substances will help you create a room that is healthy for your new child.

I suggest buying a crib that is metal with a nontoxic coating (make sure you ask the dealer), or one made of natural wood that is not covered with varnish or paint. Look for the same materials when shopping for a high chair.

Your baby will be spending a lot of time in his crib, so you want his mattress to be free of polyurethane foam, vinyl (PVC), phthalates, and chemical fire retardants. Use an organic wool mattress, which is naturally flame-retardant, and select sheets and pads made of organic cotton. This will help keep the baby's air free and clear.

The care you take in choosing room furnishings should also be applied to selecting strollers, car seats, and playpens. One good option is 100-percent polyester. While this fiber is not the best choice for clothing, when it comes to other baby items, it is a far safer option than its alternative, vinyl. Polyester cleans up well and off-gases much less than vinyl. Of course, you can also use all-natural materials, fibers, and finishes. By following these recommendations, you will go a long way toward making your child's world safe and healthy.

OUTSIDE THE HOUSE

If you're like most people, during good weather, you make the most of the outdoors and spend time on your deck or in your garden. For that reason, you should be just as diligent about keeping your outdoor areas toxin-free as you are about keeping the inside of your home safe.

A beautiful lawn can certainly make a house look nice, but you need to be aware that pesticides and even some fertilizers contain toxic chemicals such as atrazine that pose a hazard to you and your family. Look into all-natural fertilizers such as corn gluten meal, which helps reduce weeds. When cutting your grass, let the clippings remain on the lawn, as they will act as a natural compost and improve the health of the lawn. If you do decide to use a pesticide on your lawn, don't walk on it and don't let your kids or pets play on it for at least a week. If you want to keep insects away from plants, try spraying them with neem oil.

If you have a deck adjacent to your home, you may have to stain and seal it every year as a part of annual maintenance. Be careful, though, when choosing the products you use on your deck, as they can contain many of the same chemicals found in interior products. Look for nontoxic water-based paints, stains, and primers, and oil-based sealants that will not introduce harmful chemicals into your outdoor fun.

Car Smarts

To many people, their car is an extension of their home. Certainly, most of us spend a lot of time in the car, so it pays to be aware of the environment found within the car and within the garage, too.

If you're lucky enough to have a new car, and you can avoid driving it for a few days, you may want to allow the car to off-gas a bit by parking it in your driveway with the windows down. The interior of a new car contains many of the toxic chemicals found in new homes; that's what the new car smell is all about. If you have to drive your new beauty right away, keep the windows down whenever possible.

If you do some automobile maintenance yourself, be sure to perform it outside so that there is adequate ventilation for the chemicals being used. I also suggest wearing a protective mask and gloves.

If you park your car in a closed garage, it's a good idea to leave the garage door open for a few minutes after pulling the car in at night. This will allow the gas fumes to move out of the garage, rather than lingering there. If you have an attached garage, consider taking the long route around to the front door of your home, rather than walking directly from the garage into the house. This will keep fumes from getting into your living area.

Dirt, dust, and pollen settle into your car just as they settle into your home. For that reason, I suggest that you vacuum your car on a regular basis and clean it—both inside and out—with the same natural products you use in your home. This will help prevent the respiratory problems that many people suffer when dust and dirt build up.

The Downside of Golfing

Golf seems like a wholesome outdoor sport, and certainly, all the walking is wonderful for your health. Unfortunately, golf courses are kept green and beautiful through the use of chemical sprays that include toxins such as thiram and iprodione. If you love to golf, try to schedule tee times later in the day, because commercial products are usually applied to the grass early in the morning. When you get home, remove and wash your socks and golf shoes to rid them of any harmful chemicals.

CONCLUSION

It may seem an overwhelming task to eliminate the toxins from your home, but rest assured that it doesn't have to be difficult or expensive to create a more healthy environment. Begin by being aware of the many sources of toxins. As you use up your old cleaning products, replace them with more natural cleansers. They will do just as good a job as the old products, but will not fill your body with harmful chemicals. Whenever you redecorate a room or add a new piece of furniture or accessory, look for nontoxic materials. Use sealants to prevent materials from off-gassing. (Remember that you have to use the sealant only once!) As you make each modification, large or small, you will be helping your body better detoxify, repair, and rebuild. You don't have to do everything at once. Small changes in your environment can make big improvements in your well-being.

Congratulations! You have completed step sixteen on your road to outstanding health.

Remember, Health is Wealth!

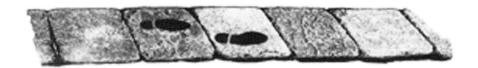

17. Household Electricity

What's your frequency?

Electricity is one of our greatest modern conveniences and one for which I am especially grateful. I think we all become acutely aware of the importance of electricity whenever a storm blows the power out and we are left without light, heat, television, computers, and sometimes even the ability to cook. Many of us are so dependent on this valuable resource that our lives stand still until power is restored.

Is all of this electricity good for us or bad for us? For that matter, is it all the same, or do different modern conveniences affect the human body to different degrees? This chapter begins by discussing the electromagnetic spectrum, which includes the different forms of energy to which we are exposed each day, both natural and man-made. It then looks at the various sources of electromagnetic energy in our environment and explores how we can use modern technology without causing harm to our health.

THE ELECTROMAGNETIC SPECTRUM

The electromagnetic (EM) spectrum is the range of all possible frequencies of electromagnetic energy—energy that comes not only from our planet but also from the rest of our solar system, and is emitted by objects in the form of electrical and magnetic waves. EM radiation is classified into the following categories, starting with the longest wavelengths and moving to the shortest: radio waves, microwaves, infrared light, the visible region that we perceive as light and color, ultraviolet light, x-rays, and gamma rays. Each type of EM radiation behaves differently and interacts with matter in different ways, depending on its wavelength. Some EM radiation is healthy for us, while some of it is not.

At one end of the spectrum are radio waves, the longest wavelengths, which are produced by astronomical bodies such as planets, comets, and stars. These frequencies are harnessed through antennae and used to transmit data. Televisions, wireless networking, and radios all use radio waves.

Microwaves are shorter than radio waves. If you use a microwave oven, you are familiar with the effects of this type of EM radiation. It heats food—not through thermal heat like conventional ovens, but by transferring energy through the food electromagnetically. Radar and cell phones also use microwave radiation.

The infrared portion of the electromagnetic spectrum has shorter wavelengths than microwaves. Like radio waves and microwaves, infrared radiation cannot be seen as light by the human eye. However, it can be felt as heat. The human body naturally radiates this type of electromagnetic energy, and many health clinics use infrared technology to help sick people get well.

The next wavelength on the spectrum is visible radiation, or light. We can see this EM radiation as it shines through the prism of our atmosphere, creating various colors. Many people enjoy a deep sense of well-being and an increase in overall health when they are exposed to the full spectrum of visible light.

Ultraviolet (UV) light is next in the electromagnetic spectrum. The wavelength of this light is shorter than the violet end of the visible spectrum, but longer than x-rays. The sun emits a large amount of UV radiation, of which there are three types. Short-wavelength UVC is potentially the most damaging, but is completely filtered out of the Earth's atmosphere and does not reach the Earth's surface. Medium-wavelength UVB is biologically active, but is mostly filtered out by the Earth's atmosphere. Relatively long-wavelength UVA accounts for about 95 percent of the UV radiation that reaches the Earth's surface. Highly energetic, UV light is *ionizing*, which means that it can detach electrons from atoms or molecules, thereby causing damage. For instance, sunburn is caused by the disruptive effects of UV radiation on skin cells. A certain amount of UV radiation, though, is necessary for the life of our planet and for human health, as well.

After ultraviolet light comes the shorter wavelengths of x-rays. X-ray radiation is emitted by celestial bodies, but is absorbed by the Earth's atmosphere without reaching the surface of the planet. X-ray radiation is also intentionally produced to take diagnostic images of the interior of the human body. However, because x-ray radiation is ionizing, it can pose a hazard to health if not used wisely and sparingly.

Finally, at the far end of the electromagnetic spectrum, are gamma waves, which have the shortest wavelength of all and are the most energetic form of light. Like X-rays, gamma rays—which are ionizing—exist in space, but are absorbed by the Earth's atmosphere. We intentionally produce gamma rays for use in the irradiation (sterilization) of foods, to kill cancer cells in radiation therapy, and in the diagnostic imaging known as PET scans. Like x-rays, gamma rays can be hazardous to your health.

Now you are a little more familiar with the electromagnetic spectrum. Some portions of the spectrum you can see as light, some you can feel as heat, and some cannot be perceived with your senses at all, but all types of electromagnetic energy affect you in one way or another. Those areas of the spectrum that are most beneficial to your health are infrared radiation, visible light, and ultraviolet rays—generally, the "middle" of the spectrum. Now, let's take a look at how some of the specific electrical devices in your life affect you by emitting various types of electromagnetic radiation, and what you can do to protect yourself.

LIGHTING

Good household and office lighting is beneficial to your health, because it allows you to perform activities such as reading without straining your eyes. I like my rooms to be well lit, so I use both ceiling and table lamps even when a room receives a lot of natural light through windows.

As you know, there are two basic types of light bulbs: incandescent and fluorescent. The "standard" light bulb that has been used in most homes for years is the incandescent bulb. It creates light by heating a filament inside the bulb. When the filament gets white-hot, it produces the light that you see. A fluorescent bulb, on the other hand, contains a mercury vapor that produces invisible ultraviolet light (UV) when the gas is excited by electricity. The UV light hits the bulb's white coating, which changes it into light that you can see. Because these bulbs don't use heat to create light, they are far more energy-efficient than incandescent bulbs.

The problem is that fluorescent light is not as healthy as incandescent light. Fluorescent lighting emits short-wave UVC radiation and a small amount of x-rays, which you now know are not within the healthy zone of the electromagnetic spectrum. In Chapter 5, I talked about how you can benefit from the positive energy emitted by the Earth and sun. By utilizing the Earth's magnetic field and the sun's natural radiation, you can help your body detoxify, repair, and rebuild cells. Fluorescent lighting, however, emits negative energy that can adversely affect people who are sensitive to it. According to an article by the National Academy of Integrative Learning, Inc., "Research in the use of light in schools has shown that cool-white fluorescent bulbs cause: bodily stress, anxiety, hyper-activity, attention problems, and other distress leading to poor learning."[1]

In Chapter 5, I mentioned that people who live in areas which receive little sunlight may benefit from full-spectrum lighting, which simulates natural outdoor lighting. Both full-spectrum incandescent and fluorescent bulbs are available.

CELL AND CORDLESS PHONES

Cell phones and cordless phones use the microwave portion of the electromagnetic spectrum to send and receive signals. As stated earlier in the chapter, the most beneficial wavelengths of electromagnetic radiation are the center wavelengths. Microwaves are not in this central zone, and currently, there is much debate over the possible dangers caused by cell and cordless phones. Studies indicate that the radiation emitted by these phones could be harmful to the brain when the devices are placed near the ear. An article printed in *Environmental Health Perspectives* stated, "We have previously shown that weak pulsed microwaves give rise to significant leakage of albumin through the blood brain barrier."[2]

I try to keep my cell phone as far away from my head as much as possible. I do not use a cell phone earpiece. Whenever, possible, I put the phone on "speaker" so that the device can be held several inches from my head. I do not use a cordless phone at all.

To make my cell phone safer to use, I have attached a diode to the back of the phone. This device converts the harmful electromagnetic field to a biologically harmless field without interfering with the phone's function. When my children are allowed to own their own cell phones, they will be instructed to use the speaker portion as much as possible and to always keep a diode on the phone.

Too Much Volume

The younger you are, the louder you want to play your music. But as you get older, unless you're in a rock band, it's very likely that you'll want to turn down the volume. Today, with so many people using iPods and wearing headsets, it is especially important to understand the very real potential for hearing loss. I have seen too many hearing problems result from high-volume broadcasting through headsets. I sound like my grandparents when I say, "Turn down that music!" But the truth is, you need to take your hearing very seriously.

MICROWAVE OVENS

As already explained, microwave ovens use the microwave portion of the electromagnetic spectrum to heat foods not by becoming hot themselves, but by

What Is an EMF?

Technically, an electromagnetic radiation field, or EMF, is any field found throughout the electromagnetic spectrum. But in popular usage, the term EMF refers to energy fields that are created by man-made objects (such as microwave ovens), and that appear to have adverse health effects.

transferring energy through the food. Although they do not deliver enough energy to be ionizing, microwave ovens emit an electromagnetic field that can extend several feet beyond the machine itself if the door of the oven has leakage problems. Therefore, these appliances can affect nearby people and pets when the oven is in operation. As explained on page 137 of Chapter 13, microwave ovens also negatively affect the food that is heated within them.

I eat nothing and drink nothing that was cooked or even heated in a microwave oven. Although I do eat in restaurants, many of which use microwave technology, I always tell the waitress ahead of time that I do not want any foods that have been microwaved.

COMPUTERS

Computers are a necessity for most of us. Whether we must use one in our profession or to communicate with people socially, to one extent or another, they are a part of our lives. Of course, like all electronic devices in the world, computers emit a form of electromagnetic radiation. This radiation is not ionizing, but it does excite electrons. The electromagnetic field generated by computers is less powerful than that generated by microwave ovens and extends only about eighteen inches beyond the machine. Therefore, it is most likely to be harmful when it is positioned very near the body. For that reason, I highly suggest that you avoid placing a laptop computer directly on your lap. Simply position the laptop on a desk or countertop so that it remains at least a few inches away and does not directly send radiation into your body. This will also place less strain on your back because you won't have to hunch over the device to use it.

It should be noted that the older box-shaped computer monitors are more of a threat in terms of emitting harmful electromagnetic radiation because they are simply greater in mass. Newer, slimmer monitors pose far less of a problem. If you have an older monitor, you may want to obtain an EMF (electromagnetic field) diode that can be placed on the computer to render the field biologically harmless.

TELEVISION

Televisions are a great invention, but as mentioned in Chapter 7, they do give off a low electromagnetic field that may be harmful. For that reason, I suggest sitting as far away from your set as you can comfortably sit without compromising your enjoyment. Like flat screen computer monitors, flat screen television sets are more body friendly because of their reduced mass. Just the same, it's best not to sit directly in front of your TV. Keep your distance, and you'll be able to enjoy television in good health for many years to come.

Digital Alarm Clocks

Consider using a battery-powered alarm clock instead of a plug-in digital alarm, which emits low EMFs. If you must use a plug-in alarm clock, keep the device on the other side of the room—not near your body.

SMOKE DETECTORS

The ability of smoke detectors to save lives and property has been documented. These alarms can alert you to a home fire while it is still possible to get your family to safety.

Be aware, though, that there are two types of smoke detectors. One type uses a small amount of radioactive material to detect smoke; the other uses a photoelectric sensor. The first type of detector emits a very low level of EMF. Although these detectors are usually installed in ceilings, and are therefore positioned several feet away from anyone standing beneath them, it seems smart to simply choose detectors that use body-friendly photoelectric sensors.

HEALTH AND ELECTRICAL FREQUENCY

Every object on the planet has an electrical frequency that can be measured by counting the number of occurrences of a repeating current flow per second. The unit of measurement used to describe electrical frequency is called Hertz (Hz). It has been discovered that the human body's general electrical frequency is within the range of 62 to 72 Hz.

It is important that any electrical device used on the body have a frequency that is similar to human frequency. I recommend that you never place upon your body an electrical device that is plugged into a wall socket—unless that device can descramble the electricity and change it into a body-friendly frequency. Electrical devices that are *not* friendly to the body include electric blankets, electric heating pads, and older-style waterbeds that have built-in heating components.

These devices have a slightly lower frequency (about 60 Hz) than what the human body naturally emits. However, it is believed that the cumulative effects can cause ill health over time.

VALERIE—A CASE STUDY

Twenty-year-old Valerie came to my clinic because she had been experiencing ringing in her ears for the last three weeks. The young lady was upset almost to the point of tears.

I examined Valerie and found no physical reason for her unusual symptom. Upon asking her a few questions about her daily life, I noticed her cell phone sticking out of her pocketbook. I asked her how long she had been using a cell phone, and she said that she had received it about a month earlier, on her birthday, and had been using it ever since. She was happy to have her own cell phone and was thrilled that it was pink, her favorite color.

I explained that cell phones generate negative frequencies and suggested that Valerie's cell phone had caused her current health problem. She looked at me with wide eyes, and I could tell she was thinking, "No more pink phone?" I told her that health is about compromise and substitution, and that if we can't or won't eliminate a harmful object, we can at least make it less harmful. I then advised Valerie to use the speaker function of her phone rather than holding it up to her ear, and also to buy an inexpensive neutralizing diode that could be placed on the phone for those times when she wanted to hold more private conversations. Whew! I spoke to Valerie the following week, and she reported that she was feeling great and still loved talking on her pink cell phone. Valerie was so excited about the results of this simple change that she also modified some of her other lifestyle habits by drinking pure water, buying healthy footwear, and using nontoxic makeup.

PROTECTING YOURSELF FROM HARMFUL ELECTROMAGNETIC FIELDS

There is a great deal of electromagnetic energy—including low-level radiation—that you can't avoid. Stray electricity surrounds you as it emanates from power lines, telephone poles, power stations, electrical transformers, etc. An article printed in *Electromagnetic Biology and Medicine* stated, "Dirty electricity is a ubiquitous pollutant. It flows along wires and radiates from them and involves extremely low frequency magnetic fields and radio frequency radiation."[3]

If you are in the market for a new house, it would make sense to choose one that avoids nearby sources of negative electrical frequency, such as electrical transformers. You can even purchase a Gauss meter, also known as a magnetometer, which will measure the level of the magnetic field in and around the house. The Environmental Protection Agency recommends a reading of 1.0 mG or lower. A reading above 2.0 mG is considered dangerous. If the reading is too high, it would make sense to search out a safer house.

If you are going to continue to live in your current home, you can't do much about the EMFs emitted by objects outside the house, but you should think about the various electric appliances inside your home. Remember, both your small and large electronic devices—computers, television sets, toasters, baby monitors, digital clock radios, and more—give off low EMFs. You probably don't want to (or can't) give up most of these modern conveniences, but there are steps you can take to make your home environment healthier. First, I suggest that you give up your microwave oven, as this poses a major health risk. Next, I suggest that you place a special diode directly on your home's circuit breaker box. This will neutralize the harmful energies emitted by your electrical wiring and appliances. This is a point-of-entry system—much like the point-of-entry water- and air-purification systems discussed earlier in the book. (See Chapters 1 and 16.) Finally, as far as possible, keep your distance from electric appliances while they are in operation.

CONCLUSION

My goal in this chapter was to simply make you aware of the many sources of harmful EMFs within your environment so that you can minimize your risk as much as possible. Because cell phones are held against your head, these now ubiquitous gadgets pose the greatest risk in terms of EMF radiation. But as you've learned, you don't have to give up modern technology to protect yourself or your family from EMFs. By taking some simple steps, you can enjoy the convenience of cell phones, computers, and many other electronic devices, and still help your body detoxify, repair, and rebuild.

Congratulations! You have just completed step seventeen on the road to superb health.

Remember, Health is Wealth!

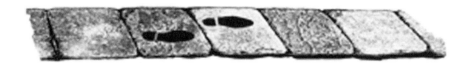

18. Nutritional Supplements

Hey, what's this green stuff?

Many people routinely take nutritional supplements of one kind or another. They may take "multi" formulas, which include both vitamins and minerals, or they may choose just minerals, just vitamins, amino acids, herbs, or a combination of several of the above. Supplements, in fact, are a multi-billion dollar industry. Some people pay more for their supplements than they do for their medications because vitamin and mineral preparations are generally an out-of-pocket expense, which means that they are not covered by health insurance. In short, people like their supplements.

Why are supplements so popular? Many people were raised with the idea that when something ails them, they should respond with a pill rather than trying to identify and correct the cause of the problem. This is one reason why people so readily embrace supplement taking. It seems like an appropriate response to a health problem, and it's easy, too—far easier than incorporating more fruits and vegetables into the diet or getting more exercise. And all these supplements just make our bodies that much stronger, right?

This chapter takes a closer look at dietary supplements. It begins by examining the best processing and packaging that results in the highest level of nutrients. It then discusses the supplements themselves and guides you in choosing those products that truly work.

PROCESSING AND PACKAGING
THAT PRESERVE NUTRITIONAL POWER

In Chapter 13, I mentioned that the greatest destroyers of the nutrients in food are air, light, and heat. The same is true of the nutrients in supplements. If supplements are heated to 125°F before they are packaged, their nutritional value is diminished. After they are packaged, exposure to further heat or to light and air can decrease their potency even more.

To ensure that you get supplements which are high in nutrients, you want to look for three features. First, you want a supplement that is either freeze-dried or processed with very low heat. This means that the nutrients were not compromised when the supplement was being processed into a powder, capsule, or tablet.

Second, you want a supplement that is packaged in an amber- or blue-colored glass bottle. The darker coloring protects the supplement from the damaging effects of light. You probably know that supplement containers often sit on the retailer's shelf for days, weeks, or even months. Therefore, light is a major concern. Many supplements are packaged in white plastic bottles, which do not adequately shield the contents from light. Dark plastic containers are a better option, but the best option is dark glass.

Third, you want to make sure that the product has been vacuum sealed, as this will keep the product fresher for a longer period of time. To ensure that no one has tampered with the contents, there should be a seal (often plastic) around the outside of the container, and a paper seal on the neck of the container, under the cap. When you puncture the paper seal you should hear a mild popping sound, signaling that the vacuum has been broken.

You may not always be able to find a supplement that has all three of the above features—a product that's freeze-dried, stored in an amber glass bottle, and vacuum sealed—but try to find a product that has as many of these features as possible. When companies bother to use amber-colored glass bottles and vacuum seals, it's a good indication that they have made a high-quality supplement whose nutrients are intact.

WHOLE FOOD-BASED SUPPLEMENTS

The best supplement you can buy is one that is food-based, meaning that it is *an actual food* rather than being created in a laboratory or extracted (isolated) from a food. This will enable your body to absorb and use it. You do not want to take an isolated nutrient or a multivitamin-and-mineral tablet that contains a group of isolated nutrients. Why? Let's say that you eat a carrot, which is full of vitamin A. Because the carrot contains other substances that help the body break the vegetable down and utilize its components, your body is able to benefit from the vitamin A. But it has been found that when the vitamin is ingested alone, without all the nutrients and other compounds found in a whole food, the body either eliminates the vitamin or stores it as a toxin. It is simply unable to recognize and utilize that solitary nutrient. Over time, a toxic situation develops. According to an article printed in *The Journal of Clinical Endocrinology and Metabolism*, "Once nutrients are isolated in tablet form, they become in all effects a pharmacological preparation. Tableting compounds may drastically influence their bioavailability and hence, influence clinical effects."[1] It is very hard, if not impossible, to duplicate in a laboratory what Nature has already created.

Fortunately, it is not necessary to duplicate Nature's work, because two of Nature's products—bee pollen and blue-green algae—contain nearly every vitamin, mineral, enzyme, amino acid, and essential fatty acid known to man. In fact, bee pollen and blue-green algae pack so much nutrition that they are often referred to as *superfoods*. Let's take a look at these two whole food-based supplements.

Bee Pollen

When bees collect pollen (seeds) from flowers, they pack the powder into granules, adding honey or nectar from their sacs. They also add digestive enzymes to prevent the pollen from germinating. The result is a true superfood that contains more than ninety-six different nutrients, including vitamins, minerals, amino acids (the building blocks of protein), polyunsaturated fatty acids, and enzymes.

Clearly, bee pollen is a nutritional powerhouse, but it also has added benefits. Some experts believe that it can help lower sensitivity to local plant pollen, which has been known to trigger allergies. It also is helpful in balancing hormones.

Bee pollen generally comes in seed form, and as mentioned earlier, is most potent when it has been freeze-dried. You can eat it as is, or you can use a rolling pin to grind up the seeds, and mix them into your daily fresh fruit or vegetable juice to create a nutrient-packed drink. You can also stir the supplement into food.

Blue-Green Algae

Blue-green algae and spirulina—which is a specific form of blue-green algae—are found in Nature, growing in the alkaline waters of lakes and ponds. Like bee pollen, these superfoods are rich in vitamins, minerals, amino acids, essential fatty acids, and many more nutrients. Blue-green algae has been found to aid digestion, enhance the health of joints and the heart, reduce inflammation in the body, and perform many other important functions. Remember, too, that blue-green algae contains chlorophyll, a substance that rebuilds and replenishes red blood cells, detoxifies the body, and boosts energy.

Blue-green algae products are generally available in tablet, capsule, or powder form. Obviously, the powder form is easiest to mix into your daily juice, but if you find only tablet form, you can easily crush it with a rolling pin so that it can be added to beverages or foods.

Adult Dosage

Because bee pollen and blue-green algae are whole foods, you can take whatever amount you want. You don't have to worry about overdosing on these wholesome products! However, be aware that these are nutrient-dense supplements, and most people are not used to this type of nutrition. Therefore, I suggest that you use the following schedule.

Start by adding one-quarter teaspoon of blue-green algae to one of your drinks every day. About every two weeks, add another one-quarter teaspoon until you have built up to a full teaspoon of algae. Once this level is achieved, start adding one-quarter teaspoon of the bee pollen to your drink as well, and increase the bee pollen amount every two weeks, just as you built up the blue-green algae. Eventually, you should be consuming about a teaspoon of the algae and a teaspoon of the bee pollen every day. (For children's dosage, see page 194.)

Some patients reported that when they started using these whole-food supplements, they felt a little warm or experienced a touch of diarrhea. This can occur because the body's detoxification process is kicked into a higher gear when you begin consuming high-quality nutrition. Be assured that these "side effects" will not last long, and that your body will benefit greatly from the supplements. I know people who consume a tablespoon or more of these products every day!

Be aware that there are whole food supplements that contain both bee pollen and blue-green algae in one product. This type of combination supplement is just fine. Simply remember to start with a small amount and build up the dosage slowly.

The Daily Value

If you look at a bottle of multivitamin-and-mineral supplements, you will see the nutrients in each "serving" expressed as a percentage of the Daily Value, or DV. The Daily Value is the amount of that nutrient which a healthy person should consume in one day based on a 2,000-calorie diet. If you are eating foods in their natural state and you take whole food-based supplements, you won't have to worry about getting your Daily Value because you'll be getting all the nutrients you require! If you take in more of a vitamin or mineral than your body needs, it will extract the right amount of nutrition from your food and eliminate the rest.

ANNE—A CASE STUDY

Anne was an elderly woman who prized her independence. She was proud of the fact that she still drove her car and could get around town on her own. She was concerned, though, that she had begun to develop various aches and pains, as well as an unsteadiness that was getting worse over time and made it necessary for her to use a cane. Her patient symptoms form included a good many checks. Anne told me that she was "into" nutrition and took a couple of supplements, so I asked her to bring everything she was taking to her next clinic appointment.

A week later, Anne came into my office with a plastic bag full of pill vials. When she dumped the contents onto the table, there must have been fifty bottles of prescription meds and over-the-counter supplements! After I picked up the bottles that had fallen to the floor, I began to review them with her. It was amazing to me that she could keep them all straight. The truth was, she couldn't.

I explained to Anne that none of her pills were doing her any good. She was confused, "How come the lady at the health store told me to take these supplements and the doctor told me to take these medications?" I asked her how long she had been feeling rather poorly, and she said for about two years. I asked her how long she had been taking all this stuff, and she replied that she'd been using them for about two years. Enough said.

I told Anne that she needed to get on the road to health and that we would take the journey together. First, I explained that she required whole food-based supplementation, but only two products: blue-green algae and bee pollen. I then called her doctor and explained that Anne needed to take a different course of action to treat her health problems. We didn't want to take Anne off the medication "cold turkey," since that could cause a mini-withdrawal. Instead, we discussed a plan that would slowly wean her off all the drugs that she did not need. I told Anne how to further detoxify her body by drinking steam-distilled water and using special showerhead filters. Anne would also switch to a diet of clean foods, which would include raw and juiced organic produce; begin a weekly fasting program; build up to taking a gentle twenty-minute walk in the early-morning sunshine, aided by her cane; use balance exercises; practice regular bowel habits; and adopt a consistent sleep schedule. In short, she would follow most of the steps described throughout this book. Anne remarked that this was all easy and fun for her as she was simply exchanging one activity, food, or product for another.

A year after Anne's first visit to my clinic, she attended a family reunion. This time, she had no aches or pains, and she didn't need her cane for balance. She glowed with health and vibrancy and was the talk of the reunion. Anne told me that it was the best day of her adult life. Her family was so impressed, in fact, that one by one, they began their own journeys on the road to health.

PROBIOTICS

Another type of supplement should be mentioned before we complete our discussion of supplement basics. First explained in Chapter 8 (see page 110), probiotics are the "friendly" bacteria that live in your body, performing a number of useful functions. Probiotics help maintain digestive health, keep potentially harmful organisms such as yeast under control, and strengthen the immune system. Foods such as yogurt, kefir, unprocessed cheese, raw unpasteurized goat's milk, and sauerkraut all provide a healthy dose of probiotics.

It is a good practice to eat probiotics-rich food in your everyday diet to maintain your body's colonies of good bacteria. If you are taking antibiotics (which kill both good and bad bacteria) or are experiencing a bacterial infection, it is truly *necessary* to either add these foods to your diet or to take probiotics in supplement form.

If you opt for probiotic supplements, look for them in capsule or powder form. Some products contain one type of bacteria, and some contain several different types. Make sure that your supplement contains at least *Lactobacillus acidophilus* and *bifidobacterium*.

Adult Dosage

I suggest that you take at least 6 billion live cultures per day. I know you are thinking that this is a lot, but it really amounts to only about three capsules, or about three-quarters of a teaspoon of powder. (For children's dosage, see page 194.)

Like blue-green algae and bee pollen, probiotics can be dissolved in juice or stirred into food. Because these supplements contain live bacteria, they usually have to be refrigerated to keep the bacteria viable.

Wheat and Barley Grass Supplements

The blue-green algae and bee pollen discussed in this chapter provide all the nutritional supplementation that most people need. But it's important to note that there are other excellent food-based supplements: wheat and barley grass. Both of these grasses are loaded with essential vitamins, minerals, and other nutrients, including antioxidants. Like blue-green algae, they are rich in chlorophyll and promote a healthy alkaline environment in the body. You can buy these supplements in tablet, capsule, or powder form, or you can juice the fresh grasses. If using the powdered supplement, slowly build up your dosage from one-quarter teaspoon to a full teaspoon, and enjoy the added benefits of high-nutrient grass along with your other food-based supplements.

SUPPLEMENTATION FOR CHILDREN

Parents routinely ask me if their children can take supplements, and the answer is a definite *yes*. Children can take the same whole food-based supplements used by adults, and can take probiotics, too. They just need to take smaller amounts.

Children's Dosage

Wait until your child is around two years of age before beginning supplementation. At that point, children are usually eating the full spectrum of solid foods. I recommend starting with one-eighth teaspoon of blue-green algae a day, mixing it into food or juice. Every couple of weeks, add another eighth of a teaspoon. Once your child is taking a half teaspoon of blue-green algae, you can introduce bee pollen, starting with one-eighth teaspoon and increasing the amount every two weeks until the child is taking one-half teaspoon. These amounts of whole food-based supplements can be used until the child is a teenager. At that point, he can take the "adult" amounts explained on page 191.

If your child is two years of age or older and suffers from a bacterial infection and/or is taking a course of antibiotics, it's a good practice to supplement his diet with probiotics. Look for a supplement that contains *Bifidobacterium infantis*, which is a gentle strain of bacteria. I suggest giving your child about 2 billion live cultures a day, which translates into one capsule or one-quarter teaspoon. Continue to supplement with probiotics until the infection has subsided or the course of antibiotics has ended.

ANGIE—A CASE STUDY

Angie was fifty-one years old and had just moved into town. When she visited my clinic, she said that for most of her adult life, she had been feeling "pretty good." During the last year, though, her spine and other joints of her body had been giving her "fits." A couple of years earlier, Angie had been diagnosed with osteoporosis. Her doctor had told her to load up on calcium pills and to make sure to drink lots of milk, and she had followed his recommendations. Unfortunately, the pain in her joints had only gotten worse.

I explained to Angie that it was not helpful to take calcium pills alone, as an isolated nutrient. Her body could not recognize the nutrient as a food and was unable to utilize it. Moreover, the milk she was drinking was pasteurized so that most, if not all, of the nutrients had been destroyed. So while Angie had been consuming lots of calcium, her body was not getting what it needed to repair and rebuild itself.

I instructed Angie to start a diet of fresh vegetable juice, to drink clean water, to incorporate some walking into her daily routine, to spend time out in the sunshine, and to take whole food-based nutritional supplementation. Gradually, Angie's bones became stronger and her spine and joint pains subsided.

Choosing and Storing Nutritional Supplements

This chapter directs you to supplements that will naturally help you enhance and maintain your health. Although I've tried to make my recommendations for choosing supplements as simple and straightforward as possible, you may find the following abbreviated guidelines helpful.

❑ Try to get most of your nutrition from your diet, but take whole food-based supplements—specifically, bee pollen and blue-green algae—on a daily basis to make sure that your body gets all the nutrients your body requires for vibrant health.

❑ Shop at a natural food store. The supplements at an ordinary grocery store are usually not 100-percent natural. Look for supplements that contain no preservatives or artificial coloring—nothing but the whole food-based supplement itself. Be especially careful to avoid ingredients and fillers to which you have a sensitivity or allergy. Usually, the supplement label will tell you if that product contains soybeans, dairy, gluten, and other ingredients that may be problematic.

❑ Buy freeze-dried supplements or supplements that have been exposed to no or only low heat. Remember that heat destroys nutrients.

❑ Make sure that the supplement is packaged in a container that protects it from the light. Amber-colored glass is the best choice.

❑ Choose products that have been vacuum sealed to preserve freshness. When you puncture the paper seal over the container, you should hear a mild popping sound indicating that the vacuum has been broken. Also make sure that the container has a tamper-proof seal.

❑ If you are taking a course of antibiotics or experiencing a bacterial infection, either supplement your diet with probiotics-rich foods such as yogurt, or take a probiotics supplement.

❑ Keep both your blue-green algae and your bee pollen supplements in a cool, dry place to help maintain the products' freshness and viability. Be sure to store probiotics as directed on the package. Most brands have to be kept in the refrigerator.

Avoiding Medication When You Can

By embracing a healthy lifestyle, you can often avoid health disorders or correct them over time. My patients were often able to use a prescribed drug for only a short period of time—just to ease their symptoms until lifestyle changes naturally corrected the problem. While they were taking the medication and afterwards, I guided them in removing the toxins from their system so that they could live drug- and toxin-free.

MEDICATIONS

Since many people take both supplements and medications—often to treat the same health disorders—it makes sense to say a few words here about medication.

I feel that medications have their place if used with commonsense. If your doctor prescribes a medication for a health problem, first ask the purpose of the medication and whether it will correct the problem or simply help control it. Also ask if there are dietary alternatives. If, for instance, you are taking the medication for high blood pressure, might a change of diet make the medication unnecessary? Inquire about side effects, too. Finally, ask how long you will have to remain on the drug and if there is a plan to help wean you off it once it has done its job.

If you do need to take a medication for a long period of time—perhaps even a lifetime—take the steps outlined in this book to assist your body in detoxification so that your cells and organs can continue to repair and rebuild. On page 193 of this chapter, I mention the importance of taking probiotics during antibiotic therapy. Also integrate other components of good health outlined in this book, including pure water, clean food, exercise, fasting, sunshine, adequate rest, and the regular elimination of waste products. All of this will help your body remain clean and strong throughout treatment with medication.

CONCLUSION

Whole food-based supplements, taken daily, help ensure that you get the nutrients you need to keep your body healthy. By eating good, clean food and taking whole food supplements, you will keep your body functioning at its optimum level and avoid the development of many health disorders. When needed, probiotic supplementation will restore your body's supply of healthy bacteria and re-establish balanced good health.

You are doing well in completing step eighteen on the road to perfect health. Remember, Health is Wealth!

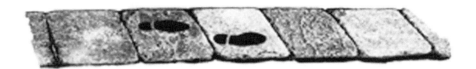

19. Integrative and Alternative Therapies

The many roads to wellness.

Many years ago, when people became ill, they would turn to a conventional medical doctor for help. After all, few or no other alternatives were available. But these days, there are as many types of healthcare providers as there are health disorders. You can see a medical doctor, who practices conventional medicine, sometimes called *allopathic medicine*, or you can see one of a number of alternative doctors and practitioners. It's all up to you.

Certainly, a growing number of people now embrace alternative therapies. The National Center for Complementary and Alternative Medicine states that approximately 38 percent of adults and 12 percent of children are using some form of CAM—treatments that are used together with standard medical care, or treatments that are used in place of standard care.[1]

This chapter is an introduction to the world of alternative healthcare treatments. It first provides some advice about choosing a supportive alternative clinic and then briefly explains the integrative and alternative therapies that can help you on the road to wellness.

WHAT ARE INTEGRATIVE AND ALTERNATIVE THERAPIES?

Before I start talking about specific therapies, it's important that you understand what the terms *integrative therapy* and *alternative therapy* actually mean.

Integrative therapy involves the use of various therapeutic techniques to address a patient's problems. The idea is that each individual is unique and that a one-size-fits-all approach is not effective. In integrative therapy, a program is developed especially for each patient's needs by combining different techniques.

The term *alternative therapy* refers to treatments that are outside the scope of conventional medical practice. This type of therapy can include nutrition and supplements, aromatherapy, hydrotherapy, chiropractic, acupuncture, homeopathy, massage, naturopathy, and more.

Always remember that the primary goals of alternative and integrative healthcare should be to address the cause of the problem—not just the symptoms. As you probably noticed, these are the same goals I discuss throughout this book. Through detoxifying, repairing, and rebuilding, you can treat a wide range of disorders and conditions. And by dealing with the cause of the problem, you not only eliminate symptoms but also lessen the risk of reoccurrence.

CHOOSING A SUPPORTIVE HEALTHCARE PROVIDER AND CLINIC

When considering an alternative health clinic or any clinic for yourself or your family, make sure that the professionals involved will give you the time and support you will need as you travel the road towards greater health. Take note of the way in which the staff treats you, starting with the very first time you call for an appointment. The staff is trained—or *should* be trained—to answer the phone in a specific way. If you find that the person who answers the phone is rude and uncaring, your healthcare visit will probably not turn out as you would have hoped. If you are not treated well on your first visit, how do you think you'll be treated after the second or third appointment?

After you have your first examination with a new healthcare provider, be sure to ask the doctor about the treatment she has in mind, such as:

❏ What is the desired outcome of my treatment?

❏ What is the overall plan for my health?

❏ How long will my treatment regimen take?

❏ How will I feel from the effects of the treatment?

❏ How expensive will my treatment be?

❏ When can I start to wean off whatever treatment I am receiving?

❏ What will be the positive and negative side effects (if any) of my treatment?

❏ How will my health benefit from the care that I receive from you?

Remember that you are not only a patient but also a consumer. Your healthcare provider should be happy to take the time needed to answer all of your questions. If she is not willing to answer your questions, do you really trust her to care for your health?

What should you do if you are disappointed by your healthcare provider or her staff? Don't feel that you have to put up with behavior that is inconsiderate or indifferent. Instead, look for competent, caring people who will work with you as a team.

COMMON ALTERNATIVE HEALTHCARE SERVICES

Alternative healthcare clinics can provide a wide range of treatments and services. Rather than focusing on individual symptoms, these practitioners take a whole-body approach to improve overall health, and also seek to help you learn about self-care so that you can better maintain health.

Some clinics expect you to stay an extended period of time—from two weeks to a couple of months. This longer stay is desired because the healthcare provider wants to start the detoxifying, repairing, and rebuilding process, and also have a chance to teach you how to take care of yourself when you get home. Other clinics don't arrange long stays, but instead offer regular visits during which they can evaluate your condition, provide treatment, and guide you in making lifestyle changes.

Below, I will first discuss some of my preferred ways of detoxifying the body. Following this, I will discuss alternative therapies that repair and rebuild health.

Detoxifying the Body

In earlier chapters of this book, I explained that poor lifestyle choices—impure water, unclean food, lack of exercise, and more—lead to the buildup of toxins in the body. This buildup also results from pollutants in the atmosphere, and even from the use of non-food-based supplements and prescription medications. One of an alternative-care provider's first jobs with any patient is to remove that toxic buildup. The following techniques are all effective means of accomplishing this.

Lymphatic Massage

Lymphatic massage is an excellent detoxification technique. As the name of this treatment implies, the practitioner massages the lymphatic channels that run along the sides of the body so that the lymph will flow more efficiently, removing toxins from tissues so that they can be eliminated. This massage is of longer duration than the shower massage that I describe on page 17 of Chapter 1.

Supervised Fast

In Chapter 3, I described the benefits of a detoxifying twenty-four-hour fast, which is adequate for most people. In the case of an individual with an advanced health condition, however, an extended supervised fast of three to seven days can be very healing. This fast usually includes only clean, pure water at the beginning and then introduces fresh juices at around day two or day three. The water begins the detoxifying process, and the juices start repairing and rebuilding the body.

Ozone Therapy

By infusing the body with ozone, which breaks down into oxygen, ozone therapy eliminates free radical formation in the body and supports the body's detoxification process. Ozone can be provided either through a tent or through an IV (intravenous) solution.

Far Infrared Sauna

Far infrared saunas use an invisible band of infrared light to provide the body with "deep heating." This, along with sweating, promotes detoxification.

You can stay in a far infrared sauna for up to an hour. The heat can get up to 190°F, but it is a dry heat. Yes, I've heard that before too, but really, this is not like a conventional sauna, which makes it so difficult to breathe that you want to escape after only a few minutes. A far infrared sauna actually heats the body from within. The air around you is warm, but not uncomfortable.

While this type of sauna is used in alternative healthcare clinics, it has the advantage of being available for use at home. The saunas simply snap together and can comfortably seat two to four people.

Chelation Therapy

Chelation therapy involves the administration of a special chelating agent, such as EDTA (ethylenediaminetetraacetic acid), which binds with and removes any heavy metals that have accumulated in the body. These metals may have been absorbed from copper in plumbing pipes, mercury tooth fillings, and aluminum in deodorants and canned goods, to name just a few possible sources. The chelating agents are delivered to the body either orally or intravenously.

Repairing and Rebuilding the Body

Once a patient has been detoxified, alternative healthcare providers sometimes suggest therapies that can further improve health by repairing and rebuilding the body. Most of the following therapies can be used to help infants, children, adolescents, adults, and seniors. Some of these therapies not only repair and rebuild, but also help detoxify.

Acupuncture

Acupuncture is an ancient technique of inserting and manipulating fine needles into specific points on the body for the purpose of relieving pain and treating various disorders. The special needles affect energy flow along energy pathways known as *meridians*.

Although this procedure sounds painful, it is really painless because the needles are so thin that they don't cut the skin like hypodermic needles, but simply separate skin pores. When inserted, they look like hairs standing up on end.

Acupuncture is a wonderful aid to repairing and rebuilding the body's channels of energy flow, and can detoxify, as well. Although it is suitable for people of any age, I recommend waiting until a child has matured a bit before utilizing this therapy for the reason that a very young child may be frightened by the needles. Electro-point stimulation—which is similar to acupuncture, but uses no needles—is a nice option for younger children.

Aromatherapy

Aromatherapy is the use of the essential oils of plants to promote relaxation, the relief of discomfort, and healing. The oils can be employed in a number of ways—added to a warm bath, used in massage, applied in a compress, or placed in a diffuser so that a vapor mist spreads throughout the room. Different oils are used for different purposes. Lavender, for instance, is effective in calming and relaxing the mind and body.

Chiropractic

Chiropractic is based upon the removal of *subluxations*—misalignments of the spinal vertebrae as well as other joints of the body. Chiropractors use their hands or a hand-held instrument to realign the joints, and thus help restore proper nerve, joint, and muscle function to the area that was compromised. The affected area is then able to detoxify, repair, and rebuild. The roots of chiropractic date back thousands of years, and the profession has been practiced in the United States for over one hundred years.

Electromagnetic Therapy

Electromagnetic therapy uses electromagnetic energy equivalent to that of the human body to correct the body's imbalances and treat a range of disorders, including chronic pain, nerve problems, asthma, bronchitis, arthritis, and more. Electromagnetic therapy improves circulation, repairs bones, speeds healing, and enhances sleep.

Homeopathy

Homeopathy uses highly diluted amounts of a remedy that, if taken in large amounts by a healthy person, would produce symptoms similar to those being experienced by the sick individual. The remedy stimulates the body's immune system and therefore build up its defenses, allowing it to better fight a current health problem or prevent future disorders. I suggest that when using homeopathy, you avoid alcohol-based remedies, especially if you are sensitive to alcohol. Since other forms are available, including distilled water-based remedies and tiny pellets that melt on the tongue, it should be no problem to find a nonalcoholic remedy.

Hydrotherapy

Hydrotherapy, which is also known as water therapy, is the external use of water to relieve pain and promote healing and well-being. The patient can be submerged in a warm or cool water bath, can perform strengthening or stretching exercises in a swimming pool, can be exposed to water in the form of steam, or can have hot or cold water applied in the form of wraps and compresses.

Massage

Massage can take many forms, and depending on its form, can have different effects. A friction massage is designed to break up fibrous tissue adhesions in the muscles, tendons, and ligaments, and to repair and rebuild the tissues. Swedish massage is intended to relax the body, but also helps in detoxification. Lymphatic massage, discussed earlier in the chapter (see page 200), stimulates the body's lymphatic system to remove toxins.

Naturopathy

Naturopathy is an integrative form of healing that is based on the body's innate ability to heal itself. Naturopathic physicians use natural remedies—water, air, sunshine, heat, food, nutritional supplements, herbal extracts, and more—to enhance the body's capacity to combat illness and maintain well-being.

Nutritional Therapy

Nutritional therapy is based on the recognition that a myriad of health problems result from poor nutrition, and that food provides the remedy necessary to obtain and maintain good health. This holistic discipline focuses on eating or eliminating particular foods, and on using nutrients for therapeutic benefit.

Reflexology

Reflexology is based on the recognition that the feet, hands, and ears are a microcosm of the entire body, and that by stimulating particular points on these areas, you can relieve pain and promote healing and wellness in other areas of the body. Reflexology works well on people of all ages, including infants. For instance, you can relax a baby before bedtime simply by placing pressure on and rubbing the soles of the feet.

Rolfing

Also called Rolf therapy, Rolfing combines deep tissue massage with stretching to break up adhesions found in the muscles, ligaments, and tendons, often as a result of injury. Rolfing also enhances posture, brings the body's structure into proper balance, improves breathing, and increases energy.

BONNIE—A CASE STUDY

Twenty-four-year-old Bonnie came to my clinic complaining of many "mysterious" aches and pains. She had already visited many doctors, and no one had been able to help her. Yet Bonnie was unsure about seeking the alternative care I offered. I reassured her, stating that together, we would take the journey back to wellness. I explained that first, I would use treatments to help her body detoxify, repair, and rebuild. Then, I would teach her how to care for herself.

I used several alternative therapies to help Bonnie feel better, including lymphatic massage, chiropractic, acupuncture, reflexology, and electromagnetic therapy. I then told Bonnie about the lifestyle changes she could make to continue the process of healing. She started by switching to clean water and food, and implementing a weekly twenty-four-hour fast. Later, as she gained confidence in this approach, she integrated the other components of good health discussed throughout this book.

Bonnie returned to the clinic for follow-up treatments as well as to report her progress, and on each visit, I learned that more of her aches and pains had disappeared. Bonnie's posture improved, her energy levels increased, her bowel habits became regular, and her mental outlook was better than ever before. She was very glad that she had chosen a commonsense way to get well.

SPECIALIZED FACILITIES

Alternative healthcare facilities differ from one another in what they offer. Some facilities provide nutritional guidance, massage, acupuncture, chiropractic services, and so on, while others offer only one type of care. For example, a holistic dentist specializes in the health of the teeth, and a holistic optometrist specializes in eye care, but always with a focus on whole-body health. Below, you'll learn a little about what these two holistic specialists have to offer.

Dental Care

Because of her whole-body point of view, a holistic dentist is concerned not only with dental care, but also with the impact that dental health and dental work have on the rest of the body. This is especially important in the handling of teeth that have been filled with amalgams, which contain the toxin mercury.

For decades, amalgam fillings—also known as silver fillings—have been used in dentistry. Yet these fillings contain mercury, a known toxin that has been linked to problems with the immune and neurological systems. For this reason, I strongly suggest that you avoid having new amalgam fillings used in your teeth. If at all possible, I also suggest that you have old mercury fillings removed and replaced with more body-friendly materials, such as porcelain inlays. This is especially important if you intend to become pregnant. The International Academy of Oral Medicine and Toxicology published an article stating, "Mercury is released from amalgam in significant quantities, that it spreads around in the body, including from mother to fetus, and that exposure causes physiological harm. A growing number of dentists, physicians, researchers, citizen activists, politicians, and regulators have come to the conclusion that the time has come to consign amalgam to the dustbin of history."[2] Just be aware that when a dentist removes mercury-containing fillings, he can actually cause more mercury to be released into the body. Make sure that your dentist takes the appropriate precautions, such as using a dental dam to prevent the accidental swallowing of fillings, and administering oxygen through the nose to keep you from breathing in mercury vapors.

If your dentist recommends a root canal, discuss the steps that will be taken to prevent the tooth from harboring bacteria once the nerve has been removed. Many dentists now fill in the empty canals with a product called EndoCal (also called Biocalex), a body-friendly paste that prevents bacteria from growing in the canals and potentially spreading throughout the body.

Eye Care

Although a holistic optometrist can perform all the functions of a regular optometrist—for instance, she can diagnose eye disorders and prescribe medications and corrective lenses—she also takes a preventive whole-body approach that seeks to address the source of any problem. For instance, when a patient has trouble seeing distant objects, a holistic optometrist will likely evaluate the person's lifestyle and offer guidelines for handling stress, implementing an eye exercise program, and perhaps using nutrition in an effort to naturally strengthen the eye and improve vision. She may even prescribe weak corrective lenses that will enable the patient to see, but not encourage a further deterioration of sight, as stronger lenses might.

Vision correction surgery has become very popular in recent years, but is not always successful. Moreover, we really do not know the long-term effects that these surgeries will have on vision and overall health. Holistic optometrists usually suggest that before surgery is considered, the patient try nonsurgical means of correcting vision problems, including eye exercises, pinhole glasses, and "sunning" the eyes. (See pages 64 and 81 for further discussion of these topics.)

Another alternative to vision-correction surgery is vision-shaping therapy (VST), sometimes called orthokeratology, or Ortho-K. Available for people with myopia (nearsightedness), this therapy involves hard gas-permeable lenses that are worn at night to actually reshape the eyes so that you can see without the use of eyeglasses or contact lenses. These lenses must be worn every night or several nights a week to maintain the eye shape necessary for good vision during the day. The downside is that these lenses are hard, and care must be taken to avoid scratching the eye when inserting and removing them.

CONCLUSION

During my years of practice, and during the years since then, it has been my experience that therapies which take the entire patient into consideration are the most effective. By treating the whole person, and by using a multi-therapy approach tailored to individual needs, alternative medicine naturally corrects root problems rather than just addressing symptoms. This relieves symptoms while enhancing overall health—and without causing side effects. Alternative healthcare professionals also seek to educate patients so that they take an active part in attaining and maintaining health. This approach makes teammates out of doctor and patient so that they can successfully work together.

You have completed step nineteen on the road to boundless health.

Remember, Health is Wealth!

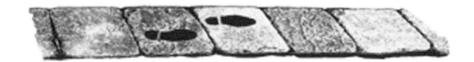

20. Treating Minor Injuries and Illness

Tending to life's minor discomforts.

No matter how well you take care of yourself, you will at some point experience a minor injury or come down with a cold, the flu, a sore throat, or nasal congestion. What can you do to treat these problems naturally and effectively? This chapter will guide you in taking care of some common injuries and disorders that can affect you and those you love.

MINOR INJURIES TO MUSCLES, LIGAMENTS, AND JOINTS

If you experience an acute injury such as the sprain of a ligament or the strain of a muscle or tendon, I recommend that you use cold water on the injury for about ten minutes, three times a day, for the first twenty-four hours, followed by twice a day for the next twenty-four hours. If the injury is not treated within that period of time, a chronic problem may result. Many people recommend applying ice to an injured body part, but I have found that liquid cold is much more effective than an ice pack. To use wet cold, soak the injured area in a cold bath, run a cold shower over the injury, or apply a cold, wet towel. This seems to penetrate deeper into the injured area than an ice pack.

Cold water is very therapeutic in that it restricts blood flow to the injured area, thereby decreasing inflammation and swelling. Blood is an excellent healer because it carries nutrients to the cells, but during the first hours of treating an injury, it's best to slow down the increased flow of blood to minimize swelling. So use cold for the first two days, and on the third and fourth days, start your shower by running warm water over the injury for five minutes, followed by five minutes of cold water. Do this twice a day. The warm water will open up the blood vessels of the injured area so that fresh blood is pumped in to start the healing phase, and the cold water will constrict the blood vessels to prevent excess blood flow. After a few minutes, your natural body temperature

ROGER—A CASE STUDY

Roger was an eighteen-year-old competitive hockey player who came to my clinic with an ankle that he had badly sprained during an afternoon game. He hobbled in with his skates on and said, "Doc, I have a big ice hockey tournament that I have to be in next week. You just have to get me better by then!" The first order of business was to remove the skate and see what was going on. Sure enough, his ankle looked like a tennis ball. I administered chiropractic to help restore some much-needed range of motion, and performed acupuncture and electromagnetic therapy to reduce the swelling. I then applied a cold pack to his ankle while my nurse wrote down the protocol described on page 207 of this chapter. Finally, I wrapped his ankle with magnets to increase stability and speed healing.

At the end of the visit, I instructed Roger to stay off the ice rink for one week. I told him that if he used the protocol and avoided skating, he would be able to play in the tournament.

Roger followed my instructions to the letter and was rewarded with daily improvements. A week after his injury, the young man laced up his skates and scored the winning goal for his team! Roger's coach was so pleased that he visited my clinic to ask how he could keep all his players healthy and active. I explained the healthy lifestyle components presented earlier in this book, and the coach shared them with his players. They responded with enthusiasm and began their individual journeys on the road to well-being.

will reopen the blood vessels. On day five, simply take a warm shower once a day. You should be feeling better at this point.

On the sixth and seventh days after the injury, start to gently stretch the injured body part under a warm shower. Hold a very gentle stretch for a few seconds while the warm water heats the affected area. For example, if you are recovering from a minor neck injury, gently tuck your chin downward, stretching the neck for a few seconds as the water warms the muscle at the back of the neck. If you are recovering from low back injury, bend forward at the waist, with one leg slightly forward and flexed, and allow the warm water to soothe your lower back for a few seconds. You can perform this daily from day six until you are fully recovered.

About a week after the injury occurs, assuming that it isn't too severe, you should be able to resume your normal activities. If you are still in pain, consider having acupuncture or chiropractic, both of which will hasten the healing process.

Many competitive athletes have a difficult time stopping their activities when they suffer from an injury. As a general rule of thumb, I recommend that— as long as the injury affects a muscle only, and you still have full range of motion—you continue with the activity, within reason, while following the advice given above. If pain restricts the range of motion, though, you should stop your exercise or activity until normal range of motion is once again achieved. If the injury has affected a joint, ligament, or tendon, stop that particular exercise until pain-free range of motion has occurred and healing is complete. A muscle receives a good supply of blood, and therefore heals faster than a ligament, a tendon, or the cartilage that creates joints.

SKIN ABRASION AND BURNS

If you have a minor skin abrasion or burn, first clean the affected area well. I suggest pouring cool water over the area and then dripping on a bit of hydrogen peroxide or—a favorite of mine—raw (unprocessed) apple cider vinegar. Both hydrogen peroxide and apple cider vinegar are good antiseptics. To begin the healing process, I suggest spreading some raw honey over the area. Raw honey has natural antibacterial powers, and has been used for centuries to treat skin problems. An article printed in the *Journal of Infection* stated, "Honey is an ideal topical wound dressing agent in surgical infections, burns and wound infections."[1]

During the day, place gauze over the area to prevent clothing from rubbing the wound and to keep dust and dirt from sticking to the honey. At night, remove the gauze so that the area is exposed to fresh air, which will promote healing. Clean and apply honey to the wound twice a day, in the morning and the evening. You should notice a steady improvement. If you do not notice an improvement within a couple of days, or if a burn is severe, consult your health-care provider.

If you wish, instead of the honey, you can use another effective healing agent: aloe vera gel. Either purchase commercial aloe vera gel or, better yet, remove it from an aloe vera plant, which you can find in most nurseries. Simply break off the end of an aloe leaf and squeeze the fresh gel over the affected area. Another option is to spread honey over the wound and then place the aloe over the honey to make it less sticky. This will prevent honey from getting on your bedding as you sleep.

ARTHRITIS

If you suffer from the pain of arthritis, you may want to try a natural topical treatment that can make you feel much more comfortable. Simply combine one teaspoon of raw apple cider vinegar with one-half teaspoon of a mixture of coconut oil and jojoba oil. Rub the resulting apple cider balm onto your aching joints as often as needed. This balm can relieve other aches and pains as well.

COLDS AND MINOR VIRAL AND BACTERIAL INFECTIONS

For most minor illnesses such as colds and flu, you'll find that a one-day water-and-lemon juice fast, as described in Chapter 3, will help the body detoxify quickly. If you are suffering from a viral infection, add a half clove of raw garlic, one-quarter teaspoon of bee propolis, or one teaspoon of raw apple cider vinegar to the water. These foods will help fight the virus. If you are suffering from a bacterial infection, probiotics will help build up your good bacteria so that they can combat the infection. Take 6 billion live cultures—about three capsules or three-quarters teaspoon of probiotics powder. Alternatively, take a teaspoon of goat's milk yogurt, goat's milk, raw cheese, kefir, or sauerkraut, all of which are rich in friendly bacteria.

On the second day of the illness, in addition to the lemon water and the antiviral or antibacterial foods, drink juiced fruits and take whole food-based supplements as described in Chapter 18. If you get hungry, drink fruit smoothies made in your blender. This will provide nutrients and fiber without taxing your body.

On the third day, you should be feeling close to normal. Resume your standard healthy diet, complete with whole food-based supplements, and continue with the antiviral or antibacterial products until you feel 100-percent well.

To determine whether your infection is bacterial or viral, note your symptoms. Generally, a bacterial infection produces little or no fever; a phlegm-producing cough; and a cloudy discharge from the nose. A viral infection produces a fever; a dry, hacking cough with little or no phlegm or mucus; and a clear discharge from the nose. With some infections, you may have symptoms of both types of infection. When this occurs, feel free to take both antibacterial and antiviral foods. If you are not noticeably better within three days, consult your healthcare provider.

Soothing a Sore Throat

When you have a sore throat, pour a teaspoonful of raw honey onto a spoon and allow the honey to drip onto the painful area. The honey will soothe your throat and also help reduce inflammation through its antibacterial properties.

NASAL CONGESTION

If you are suffering from nasal congestion, perhaps as the result of a cold, mix one drop of peppermint oil with one-eighth teaspoon of combined coconut and jojoba oil. Rub the mixture on the side of your nose, and it will help you breathe more easily.

A Neti Pot is another great way to relieve nasal congestion. Originating in India, this device looks like a little teapot. To irrigate your nasal passages, first fill the pot with clean room-temperature water. Tilt your head to the right side over a sink or bathtub, and use the Neti Pot to pour the water into your left nostril. The water will flush out your nasal passages and flow out of your right nostril. (I know this sounds weird, but it's not at all upsetting or painful.) Blow your nose to eliminate any remaining water or mucus. Now tilt your head in the opposite direction and pour the water into your right nostril. Blow your nose again, and you're done. This may be used along with the peppermint oil therapy described above.

The Neti Pot is great for colds and sinus infections and can be used on a daily basis to prevent nasal infection. If you suffer from a sinus infection, with symptoms such as nighttime coughing, headache, facial pain, and/or asthma, try adding about one-eighth teaspoon of sea salt to the water in the Neti Pot. The sea salt may burn slightly, so go very easy with it.

FEVER

The purpose of a fever is to raise the body's temperature so that it can better kill the infectious organisms that are attacking your body. Therefore, a fever is Nature's way of protecting you. Since a fever can be quite uncomfortable, however, I do offer two suggestions for lowering your temperature.

When you're suffering from a fever of 100°F or less, take a cool bath to lower your temperature. When you get out of the bath, try rubbing a mixture of peppermint oil, jojoba oil, and coconut oil on your chest. (About two drops of peppermint oil along with one-quarter teaspoon of mixed jojoba oil and coconut oil.) This will contribute toward lowering the fever and also provide a nice cooling sensation.

When your fever climbs between 101°F and 102°F, it is time to be more aggressive. Continue with the cool baths and peppermint oil rub, but also add a room-temperature enema. Room-temperature enemas are an effective fever-lowering technique that is suitable for adults and children over the age of six. Although this may not sound cooling, consider the fact that room temperature is much cooler than your internal temperature of 98.6°F. The procedure is simple, too. Fill a rubber enema bag with one to two pints (two to four cups) of clean, room-temperature water. While sitting on a toilet or kneeling on all-fours in a bathtub, place the end of the hose in the rectum, and lift the bag higher than the body. Gravity will naturally cause the water to flow from the bag into the colon.

As the water enters the colon, you will feel a strong urgency to move your bowels. At this point, remove the end of the hose and allow the bowel movement to occur. If you decide to use a tub, remember to put non-skid mats on the bathroom floor so that you won't slip when dashing from the bathtub to the toilet!

If your temperature rises above 103°F, continue with the above protocols, but also contact your doctor.

As mentioned above, I do not suggest enemas for children under the age of six because the lining of a young child's colon is too delicate. Before the age of six, lower a child's fever with cool baths and sips of cool water. (For information on treating sick infants, see the discussion that begins below.)

A colonic is different from an enema in that it uses more water. This reaches more of the colon, but also puts more stress on that portion of the digestive tract. Therefore, I do not recommend a colonic unless you have an advanced disease condition. When your objective is to lower a fever, a simple enema will be safe and effective.

Whenever you use an enema, be aware that you are flushing out good bacteria along with bad. Therefore, after the enema, make sure you eat some yogurt or other probiotics-rich food to replace the friendly bacteria that you've removed. Probiotics supplements can also be used.

Finally, keep in mind that I suggest the enema only to lower fever—not to promote regularity or to relieve constipation. If you experience constipation when you're ill, see the discussion below.

CONSTIPATION

In Chapter 8, I discussed the importance of keeping bowel movements regular by eating fresh whole foods, using colon massage, and following a generally healthful lifestyle. When you are not feeling well, though, the elimination system tends to relax, which can lead to constipation. This is one reason why I suggest a diet of lemon and water plus fresh juices when you're sick.

If you do experience constipation during an illness, you may need a little help in getting your system moving again. Twice a day, add a tablespoon of olive oil or aloe vera juice to a glass of pure water or fresh juice, and drink it down. This should make your system function properly again. If your system needs a further boost, grind up a banana and a pitted prune in the blender, and enjoy a banana-prune smoothie. If you tend to experience constipation even when you're not ill, please turn to Chapter 8 for a more complete discussion of bowel health.

INFANT ILLNESS

If your infant is being breast-fed and has a fever or an infection, give him a cool (not cold) bath along with a sip of water, followed by breast-feeding at normal feeding times. If you pump your milk, once a day, put probiotics (about one billion live cultures, or one-eighth teaspoon) in your milk before giving it to your child. Another option is to take one-quarter teaspoon of probiotics yourself so that the good bacteria will be delivered to your infant via your milk.

If you do not breast-feed your child, I suggest obtaining breast milk from a breast milk bank so that your child can benefit from its disease-protective antibodies. If this is not an option, once a day, add one-eighth teaspoon of probiotics powder to your child's formula. If you are due to give birth and do not plan to breast-feed, consider pumping your milk and freezing it soon after your child's birth. It will come in handy if your infant becomes ill.

Another good way to help your infant when he is experiencing a fever is to mix a little peppermint oil with jojoba and coconut oil, as described on page 210, and use it to massage your child's lymphatic glands. To perform this massage, run your fingertips along the sides of your child's neck just below the earlobes and work down to the collarbone. Pick up the massage again in the armpits, run your fingertips down the sides of the body to the waist, and then move into the groin area and down the inside of the thighs to the knees. Do this twice each day, morning and evening, until the fever comes down.

If your infant's fever reaches 102°F, consult with your doctor.

CONCLUSION

When you or a family member experiences a minor illness, remember that your body has the ability to detoxify, repair, and rebuild itself. This doesn't mean that you should ignore your illness. Rather, it means that you should adjust your diet to help your body fight infection and regain health. If you have experienced a minor injury, judicious natural therapeutic procedures will aid your body in healing so that you can resume your normal activities within a few days.

Congratulations. You just completed step twenty on the road to stupendous health. Remember, Health is Wealth!

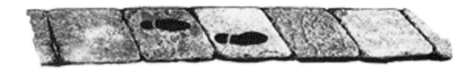

21. Putting It All Together

That was easy!

Throughout this book, I have presented a wealth of recommendations for creating physical, mental, emotional, social, and spiritual health. Now, you may be wondering how you can pull it all together into a practical daily routine. That's what this chapter is all about. I will start with your morning exercise routine and shower, and continue throughout the day until you retire at night. By the end of this chapter, you will understand how easy it is to incorporate my recommendations into a healthy lifestyle.

YOUR MORNING EXERCISE AND SHOWER ROUTINE

Try to take your twenty-minute walk in the early morning sun, breathing deeply as you walk. Temperature permitting, expose as much of your skin as possible so that you can benefit from the sun's healing rays. Three times a week, upon returning home, perform your body-weight exercises—squats, toe-raises, curl-ups, push-ups, door pull-ups, and press-ups—as well as your stretches and balance exercise. (See pages 61 to 68 in Chapter 4 for a full discussion of these exercises.)

After you have completed your exercise routine, take a nice, warm shower. (See page 16 of Chapter 1.) Be sure that the water has been purified through a point-of-entry filter and/or a special showerhead filter. Don't forget to massage your lymphatic glands using a natural coconut-based soap. Finish up your shower with a minute or so of cool water to enhance your circulation. Finally, gently rub your body with a loofah sponge or coarse towel, which will remove dead skin cells so that your skin can more easily detoxify.

As you go through your morning hygiene routine, remember to use gentle, natural, toxin-free products, as described in Chapter 14. Coconut-based soaps and shampoos, jojoba- and coconut-oil skin moisturizers, natural aluminum-free deodorants, fluoride-free toothpastes, all-natural shaving creams, and organic makeup will help you look great without burdening your body with harmful toxins.

When you finally get dressed, your best option is cotton clothing—preferably organic. At the very least, wear cotton underwear. Because undergarments are pressed directly against your body, it's important for them to be both pure and breathable so that moisture doesn't build up on your body. (See Chapter 15 to learn about other good fibers.)

BREAKFAST

Breakfast time gives you an opportunity to start your day right by meeting many of your daily nutritional requirements. I suggest that you include a glass of freshly made juice—at least eight ounces of different fruit juices. A great combination is a mixture of orange, pineapple, and strawberries. This is delicious! Use any or all of the fruits you love—grapes, grapefruit, berries, and more.

Breakfast time is also a great opportunity to take blue-green algae and bee pollen, two whole food-based supplements which will help ensure that you get all the nutrients you need each day. (See page 190 of Chapter 18 for details.) I suggest that you swirl these supplements into your morning juice. Other possible additions to your juice include a tablespoon of oat bran so that you're sure to get the fiber you need to stay regular; a teaspoon of raw apple cider vinegar, which will help your body detoxify, break up any acidic crystals that have formed in your joints, and fight viruses and parasites; and/or a teaspoon of olive, flaxseed, or coconut oil, which will enhance your skin, help your brain operate at optimum capacity, and lubricate your joints.

After you drink your juice, you can prepare your other breakfast foods, which can include natural granola cereal, toast with dairy butter or nut butter, and perhaps an egg. As discussed earlier in the book, I like to boil several eggs on the weekend and keep them in the refrigerator so that I can enjoy prepared eggs all week. (See page 27 of Chapter 2 for information about the benefits of eggs.) Just be sure to wait at least ten to fifteen minutes after finishing your juice before you eat solid foods so that your digestive acids and enzymes aren't diluted when you need them. To get the most out of your diet, you need your enzymes and acids working at full-strength during meals.

LUNCH

You may want another glass of fresh juice at lunchtime. Another good option is to place watermelon in a blender (not a juicer), with seeds intact. This watermelon beverage will provide more fiber than juice—which usually is fiber-free—and will also offer seeds, which are wonderful for your hormonal system. However, both juices and whole-fruit smoothies are high in nutrition.

Try to include a little protein (meat, beans, legumes, or nuts); some whole grains (oats, wheat, barley, millet, flax, or rice); and a fruit or vegetable, whether juiced or eaten whole, in your lunch menu. It's also good to get in some dairy, preferably in the form of goat yogurt or kefir, both of which are loaded with friendly bacteria. Don't include meat in every lunch, as it should be limited to three meals a week. If you like, top it all off with a healthy dessert.

It may seem like a tall order to include all of the above elements in a lunch, but it really isn't. A healthy midday meal might include a small salad composed of greens and beans (kidney or garbanzo beans, for instance) with a dressing of olive oil, raw honey, raw apple cider vinegar or lemon juice, and raw garlic; a multigrain bagel topped with almond butter; and a small serving of yogurt mixed with some diced fruit. Another option would be a blended watermelon drink, a hard-boiled egg, a piece of whole-grain bread or muffin, and a handful of almonds.

These are ideal menus for just about everyone, including children, adults, athletes of all ages, and seniors. They combine foods from every food group to help ensure that you are meeting all your nutritional requirements, including your need for fiber.

Clean, Pure Water

Throughout the day, drink clean, pure water that has been stored in glass or polycarbonate bottles. (See Chapter 1 for more complete information on water.) You may want to squirt some lemon juice into the water, as this will make the beverage a more effective detoxifier. Do not, however, sip water during a meal, as this can hamper digestion by diluting your digestive acids and enzymes.

DINNER

Dinner is a great opportunity to include a few more veggies. You can eat them whole—ideally in a salad—or you can juice them. If you choose a salad, use a natural dressing made of olive oil, raw apple cider vinegar or lemon juice, raw garlic, and raw honey. If you opt for juicing, use an assortment of vegetables and, to sweeten things up, add an apple or a couple of carrots. Remember, though, that you should strive for at least one salad a day because the fiber in the whole veggies will help you stay regular.

With your evening salad or vegetable juice, choose dishes that provide other food groups, such as proteins and whole grains. Whole grain pasta, brown rice, fish, homemade pizza, and lasagna are all good choices. I personally enjoy eating traditional breakfast foods such as whole grain pancakes, waffles, French toast, and eggs for dinner. Perhaps you long for an old-fashioned meal like chicken, mashed or baked potatoes, and corn on the cob. That's fine; just be sure to limit your meat, poultry, and fish to three times a week, and to use organic foods whenever they are available. Also remember to use cookware, plates, and bowls made of natural materials. Glass, stoneware, and ceramic cookware is best. (See Chapter 13 for details.)

Although good nutrition is a big part of your dinnertime, don't forget the social and spiritual aspects, which are also important. The evening meal is my personal favorite because my whole family is together, and we can share thoughts and stories. Take advantage of this time. Turn off the TV, thank God for all his blessings, and enjoy life's precious moments.

After each meal, don't forget to brush your teeth and/or use a Water Pik-type instrument to remove food particles. I know that sounds all too obvious, but there are many people who do not brush their teeth after meals. Chapter 14 will guide you in choosing natural dental-care products. (See page 153.)

Fasting

Although you should plan to have three sound meals on most days, once a week, I strongly suggest following a twenty-four-hour fast. This will allow your body to detoxify, repair, and rebuild. (For more information on fasting, see Chapter 3.)

BEDTIME

Before you retire for the night, take some time for yourself to relax and reflect upon your day. Think positive thoughts about your dreams and plans for the future. Talk to God, and spend a few minutes reading an inspirational book. This routine will help rid your mind of the day's cares and give you a positive outlook so that you can enjoy a good night's sleep. Through experimentation, you will find what works best for you. Remember that for optimum health, you should sleep from six to nine hours a night.

Make your bedroom conducive to sleep by keeping it dark and quiet. Just as important, ensure that your bedroom is a healthy place to spend the night. Keep electronic devices like TVs and digital alarm clocks in the corner of the room, as far away from you as possible. Choose cotton sheets—organic, if possible—and use an allergy-free mattress cover and a wool pillow to prevent dust mites from turning your bed into their bed. Open the window a crack to let in some fresh air. Wear loose-fitting clothing or nothing at all. All of these steps will help your body detoxify, repair, and rebuild while you enjoy a pleasant night's sleep. (For more tips on sleeping, see Chapter 7.)

A CASE STUDY

I had a patient whom I had known for a long time. He always seemed to be in good health, but he was concerned that his health might not last forever. I suggested that he drink pure water, eat organic whole foods—in short, that he follow the recommendations provided in this book. But my patient had a hectic schedule and didn't feel he had the time for healthy meals, exercise, adequate rest, and the other components of a wholesome life. While it made sense to him that others should get out in the sunshine for an early morning walk, that wasn't for him. He had responsibilities.

For a while, my patient was fine. Then one day, he woke up and realized that he was always tired, even when he'd had a full night's sleep. He was experiencing aches and pains that he hadn't felt before. He got on the bathroom scale and saw that he had lost several pounds, and it wasn't because he had been exercising. His tight schedule just didn't allow him time to eat—or so he told himself. His usual zest for life had wilted away. At lunchtime, when he had to lie down because he was so exhausted, it occurred to him that if he remained on his current path, he wouldn't be able to continue what he enjoyed doing most—helping other people.

My patient decided it was time to take control of his health. He started by drinking clean water and improving his diet. As he felt better, he began exercising. He implemented a once-a-week fast and started to follow a consistent daily schedule of exercise, meals, working, and sleeping. He improved his social relationships and deepened his communication with God. Over time, in fact, he incorporated all the suggestions found in this book into his lifestyle. It really wasn't difficult, he said. It just meant replacing old habits with new, better ones.

As days turned into weeks, my patient began to feel better than ever before. Now, he plans to live to be one hundred years old and stay as vibrant as he is today. Moreover, his life is full of joy because he is helping others achieve their own health goals.

The patient I'm describing is me. For years, I thought I was too busy to take care of my own well-being. Only when I became run-down did I realize that I had to make time for a healthier lifestyle—and the rewards have been great. Now, I have the energy I need to live life, and the good health that allows me to enjoy every moment of it.

CONCLUSION

Like every journey in life, the journey to health begins with a single step. You took that first step when you opened this book, and by now, I hope you have traveled far along the road to well-being. Remember that the goal of each stride is to make your body better able to detoxify, repair, and rebuild. While some of the steps you take may be challenging, this chapter has shown you that there are also a lot of *simple* ways to improve your health. It's really easy to drink clean water; to select clean, whole foods; and to incorporate some gentle exercise into each day. You don't have to do everything at once, either. Over time, you can make additional changes in your life to ensure that you and your loved ones enjoy the greatest riches of all—vibrant health.

Remember, Health is Wealth!

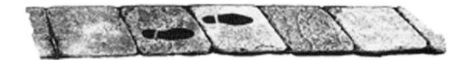

Conclusion

It has been a real pleasure walking beside you on your journey to health. It is my sincere hope that you will adopt many of the recommendations offered in these pages, for I am confident that if you do, you will be able to correct many (if not most) of your health problems and enjoy true wellness, now and for many years to come. Although my suggestions have been numerous, they boil down to less than two dozen simple steps:

❑ Drink clean, pure water and shower and bathe in clean water, as well.

❑ Eat organic whole foods, enjoying them raw or lightly cooked.

❑ Drink homemade juices—both fruit and vegetable.

❑ Supplement your diet with whole food-based supplements. Blue-green algae and bee pollen will help ensure that you get all the nutrients you need on a daily basis.

❑ Fast once a week for twenty-four hours.

❑ At least three times a week, for twenty to thirty minutes, include gentle exercise in your daily routine. Walking, body-weight exercises, and balance exercises are all important. As you exercise, remember to breathe deeply.

❑ Get twenty minutes of sunlight at least three times per week, either in the early morning or in the late afternoon.

❑ Pay attention to your standing, sitting, and sleeping posture. Good posture yields good health.

❑ Get from six to nine hours of sleep per night.

❑ Have regular daily bowel movements so that toxic wastes do not accumulate in your body.

❏ To enhance your mental and emotional health, read something educational and uplifting each day.

❏ To maintain your emotional well-being, find something that you enjoy doing, someone that you enjoy loving, and something that you can anticipate with joy.

❏ To improve your social well-being, develop positive and affirming friendships.

❏ To develop your spiritual life, spend time alone with God.

❏ Use natural cookware—glass, stoneware, or ceramic, whenever possible—and serve your food on natural dishes.

❏ Use natural, chemical-free cosmetics and personal hygiene products.

❏ Whenever possible, wear cotton clothing—preferably organic.

❏ Furnish your home with natural materials that don't add toxins to your environment, or use natural sealants to keep materials from off-gassing toxins. Also use natural, chemical-free cleaning products.

❏ Take steps to protect yourself from harmful electromagnetic fields.

I am reminded of a quote from Thomas Edison: "The doctor of the future will give no medicine but will interest his patients in the care of the human frame, in diet, and in the cause and prevention of disease." With this book in hand, you can be your own best doctor. God bless you.

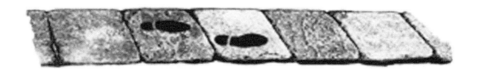

References

Chapter 1. Water

1. C. Richard Cothern, William A. Coniglio, and William L. Marcus. "Estimating Risk to Human Health." *Environmental Science Technology* 20, No. 2 (1986): 111–116.

2. Natural Resources Defense Council. "Bottled Water: Pure Drink or Pure Hype." Retrieved from www.nrdc.org/water/drinking/bw/chap1.asp.

3. Mark R. Cullen and Hugh S. Taylor. "Plastics That May Be Harmful to Children and Reproductive Health." *Environment and Human Health* (2008). Retrieved from www.ehhi./org/reports/plastics/ehhi_plastics_report_2008_pdf.

4. Cristina M. Villanueva, et al. "Bladder Cancer and Exposure to Water Disinfection By-Products Through Ingestion, Bathing, Showering, and Swimming in Pools." *American Journal of Epidemiology* 165, No. 2 (2007): 148–156.

5. Q.Q. Tang, et al. "Fluoride and Children's Intelligence: A Meta-Analysis." *Biological Trace Elements Research Journal* 126, No. 1-3 (Winter 2008): 115–120.

6. R.D. Morris, et al. "Chlorination, Chlorination By-Products, and Cancer: A Meta-Analysis." *American Journal of Public Health* 82, No.7 (1992): 955–963.

7. Evert Nieboer, et al. "Health Effects of Aluminum: A Critical Review With Emphasis on Aluminum in Drinking Water." *Environmental Review* 3 (1995): 29–81.

8. A. Bernard, et al. "Lung Hyperpermeability and Asthma Prevalence in Schoolchildren: Unexpected Associations with the Attendance at Indoor Chlorinated Swimming Pools." *Occupational and Environmental Medicine* 60 (2003): 385–394.

Chapter 2. Food

1. Christine McCullum-Gomez, Charles Benbrook, and Richard Theuer. "The First Step: Organic Food and a Healthier Future." The Organic Center (March, 2009). Retrieved from www.organic-center.org/reportfiles/Ex_Sum_pdf.

2. Isabelle Baldi, et al. "Neurodegenerative Diseases and Exposure to Pesticides in the Elderly." *American Journal of Epidemiology* 157 (2003): 409–414.

3. Han Ayden. "Soy: The Hormone Destroyer." Retrieved from www.scribd.com/doc/1013064/Soy-The-Hormone-Destroyer.

4. Erik Lykke, et al. "The Association Between Duration of Breastfeeding and Adult Intelligence." *The Journal of the American Medical Association* 287, No. 18 (May 2002): 2365–2371.

5. P.M. Clifton, J.B. Keogh, and M. Noakes. "Trans Fatty Acids in Adipose Tissue and the Food Supply are Associated with Myocardial Infarction." *The Journal of Nutrition* 134, No. 4 (April 2004): 874–879.

6. John McLachlan. "Environmental Signaling: What Embryos and Evolution Teach Us About Endocrine Disrupting Channels." *Endocrine Reviews* 22, No. 3 (2001): 319–341.

7. Evert Nieboer, et al. "Health Effects of Aluminum: A Critical Review With Emphasis on Aluminum in Drinking Water." *Environmental Review* 3, (1995): 29–81.

8. H.J. Roberts. "Aspartame Disease: A Possible Cause for Concomitant Graves' Disease and Pulmonary Hypertension." *Texas Heart Institute Journal* 31, No. 1 (2004): 105.

Chapter 3. Fasting

1. Krista A. Varady and Marc K. Hellerstein. "Alternate-Day Fasting and Chronic Disease Prevention: A Review of Human and Animal Trials." *American Journal of Clinical Nutrition* 86, No. 1 (July 2007): 7–13.

Chapter 4. Movement and Exercise

1. Miriam E. Nelson, et al. "Physical Activity and Public Health in Older Adults: Recommendation from the American College of Sports Medicine and the American Heart Association." *Journal of Circulation* 116, (2007): 1094–1105.

2. A. William Evans. "Functional and Metabolic Consequences of Sarcopenia." *Journal of Nutrition* 127, No. 5 (May 1997): 998S–1003S.

3. Arthur Jones. "The Colorado Experiment." *IronMan* 32, No.6 (September 1973) Retrieved from www.musclenet.com/coloradoexperiment.htm.

4. "Why You Should Avoid Synthetic Hormones for Menopause Treatment." *MicroNutra Health Journal* (August 28, 2008). Retrieved from www.micronutra.com/journal/menopause/why-you-should-avoid-synthetic-hormones-for-menopause-treatment.

5. I. Leibovitch and Y. Mor. "The Vicious Cycling: Bicycling Related Urogential Disorders." *European Urology* 47, No. 3 (2005): 277–286.

6. Carl T. Hall, "A Genuine Feel-Good Story: Sex May Help Prevent Prostate Cancer." *San Francisco Chronicle* (April 7, 2004).

Chapter 5. Sunlight

1. Kathleen M. Egen, Jeffrey Asosman, and William J. Blot, "Sunlight and Reduced Risk of Cancer: Is the Real Story Vitamin D?" *Journal of the National Cancer Institute* 97, No. 3 (2005): 161–163.

2. The American Academy of Family Physicians. "Seasonal Affective Disorder" (March 1, 2000) Retrieved from www.aafp.org/afp/20000301/1541/ph.html.

3. The Psoriasis Association. "Ultraviolet Light Therapy" (August 28, 2008) Retrieved from http://www.psoriasis-association.org.uk.

4. Cedric F. Garland, Frank C. Garland, and Edward D. Gorham. "Could Sunscreens Increase Melanoma Risk?" *American Journal of Public Health* 82, No. 4 (April 1992): 614–615.

Chapter 6. Posture

1. M.A. Adams and W.C. Hutton. "The Effect of Posture on the Role of the Apophysial Joints in Resisting Intervertebral Compressive Forces." *Journal of Bone and Joint Surgery* (BR) 62-B, No. 3 (1980): 358–362.

2. Bert H. Jacobson, Ali Boolani, and Doug B. Smith. "Changes in Back Pain, Sleep Quality, and Perceived Stress After Introduction of New Bedding Systems." *Journal of Chiropractic Medicine* 8, No. 1 (March 2009): 1–8.

3. N. Shakoor and JA Block. "Walking Barefoot Decreases Loading on the Lower Extremity Joints in Knee Osteoarthritis." *Arthritis & Rheumatism* 54, No. 9 (September 2006): 2923–2927.

Chapter 7. Sleeping and Resting

1. Ellen Frank, Jodi M. Gonzalez, and Andrea Fagiolini."The Importance of Routine for Preventing Recurrence in Bipolar Disorder." *American Journal of Psychiatry* 163 (June 2006): 981–985.

2. Giovanni Costa. "The Impact of Shift and Night Work on Health." *Applied Ergonomics* 27, No. 1 (February 1996): 9–16.

3. Ellen T. Kahn-Green, et al. "The Effects of Sleep Deprivation on Symptoms of Psychopathology in Healthy Adults." *Journal of Clinical Sleep Medicine* 8, No. 3 (April 2007): 215–221.

4. Baylor College of Medicine Public Affairs. "Magnetic Therapy Reduces Pain in Post-Polio Patients." (November 3, 1997) Retrieved from www.bcm.edu/news/ item/ .cfm?newsID=255.

5. United States Environmental Protection Agency. "Label Instructions Tightened on Flea & Tick Control Products for Pets." (November 2002) Retrieved from www.epa.gov/pesticides/factsheets/hartzq_a.htm#adverse.

Chapter 8. Bowel Health

1. J.H. Cummings, et al. "Influence of Diets High and Low in Animal Fat and Bowel Habit, Gastrointestinal Transit Time, Fecal Microflora, Bile Acid, and Fat Excretion." *Journal of Clinical Investigation* 61, No. 4 (April 1978): 953–963.

2. T.E. Roy. "Antibiotics and Iatrogenic Disease." *Pediatrics* 22, No.1 (July 1958): 164–170.

Chapter 9. The Mind

1. George P. Chrousos and Philip W. Gold. "A Healthy Body in a Healthy Mind—and *Vice Versa*—The Damaging Power of 'Uncontrollable' Stress." *Journal of Clinical Endocrinology & Metabolism* 83, No. 6 (1998): 1842–1845.

2. Stephen G. Post. "Altruism, Happiness and Health: It's Good to Be Good." *International Journal of Behavioral Medicine* 12, No. 2 (2005): 66–77.

Chapter 10. Building an Emotionally Satisfying Family Life

1.Barbara H. Fiese. "Routines and Rituals: Opportunities for Participation in Family Health." *Occupation, Participation and Health* 27, No. 4 (Fall 2007). Retrieved from www.otjronline.com/view.asp?rID=24568.

Chapter 11. Social Relationships

1. Jeffrey A. Simpson, et al. "Attachment and the Experience and Expression of Emotions in Romantic Relationships: A Developmental Perspective." *Journal of Personality and Social Psychology* 92, No. 2 (2007): 358.

Chapter 11. The Soul

1. Jeff Stanley. "The Three-Fold Love of God: Part 1—God's Love for Us." *Biblical Research Journal* (January/February 1994):1. Retrieved from www.biblicalresearchjournal.org.

Chapter 13. Preparing, Storing, and Eating Your Food

1.Richard Quan, et al. "Effects of Microwave Radiation on Anti-infective Factors in Human Milk," *The Journal of Pediatrics* 89, No. 4 (April 1992): 667–669.

2. Takashi Sugimura. "Nutrition and Dietary Carcinogens." *Carcinogenesis* 21, No. 3 (March 2000): 387–395.

3. M.H. Gault and L. Purchase. "Would Decreased Aluminum Ingestion Reduce the Incidence of Alzheimer's Disease?" *Canadian Medical Association Journal* 145, No. 7 (1991): 793–804.

Chapter 14. Beauty and Hygiene

1. Rebecca Sutton. "Adolescent Exposures to Cosmetic Chemicals of Concern." Environmental Working Group (September 2008) Retrieved from www.ewg.org/ reports/teens.

2. Mohammed Wadaan and Mohammed Mubarak. "Skin Lesions Induced by Sodium Lauryl Sulfate (SLS) in Rabbits." *Journal of Medical Sciences* 5, No. 4 (2005): 320–323.

3. Daniel Almajuer, et al. "Health Hazard Evaluations." National Institute for Occupational Safety and Health (May 1992) Retrieved from htt://www.cdc.gov/niosh/hhe/reports/pdfs/1989-0138-2215.pdf.

4. Use of Household Cleaning Products with Antibacterial Ingredients Did Not Reduce Symptoms of Infection." *Annals of Internal Medicine* 140, No. 5 (March 2005): 1–30.

5. Rose Marie Williams. "Makeup's Ugly Secrets." *Townsend Letter.* Retrieved from www.townsendletter.com/FebMar2006/envirohealth0206htm.

Chapter 15. Clothing

1. C.C. Hsieh and P. Trichopoulos. "Breast Size, Handedness, and Breast Cancer Risk." *European Journal of Cancer* 27, No. 2 (1991): 131–135.

2. R.D. Phillips, et al. "Modification of High-Heeled Shoes to Decrease Pronation During Gait." *Journal of the American Podiatric Medical Association* 81, No.4 (1991): 215–219.

3. Keith Rome, Den Hancock, and Daniel Poratt. "Barefoot Running and Walking: The Pros and Cons Based on Current Evidence." *New Zealand Medical Journal* 121, No. 1272 (April 2008): 109.

Chapter 16. Household Cleaners and the Home Environment

1. "Indoor Air Pollution Fact Sheet." American Lung Association (August 1999). Retrieved from www.lungsusa.org/site/pp.usp?c=dvluk900Eandb=35381.

2. Brenda Eskenazi. "A Study of the Effects of Perchlorethylene Exposure on the Reproductive Outcomes of Wives of Dry-Cleaning Workers." *American Journal of Industrial Medicine* 20, No. 5 (Jan 2007): 593–600.

3. Judy Waytiuk. "Piling It On: Are Your Carpets Harboring Health Hazards?" *The Environmental Magazine*. Retrieved from www.emagazine.com/view?414.

Chapter 17. Household Electricity

1. Laurence D. Martel. "Light: An Element in Ergonomics of Learning." National Academy of Integrative Learning, Inc. Retrieved from www.intellearn.org.

2. G Leif, et al. "Nerve Cell Damage in Mammalian Brain after Exposure to Microwaves from GSM Mobile Phones." *Environmental Health Perspectives*, Vol. 111 (2003).

3. Magda Havas. "Electromagnetic Hypersensitivity: Biological Effects of Dirty Electricity with Emphasis on Diabetes and Multiple Sclerosis." *Electromagnetic Biology and Medicine* 25, (2006): 259–268.

Chapter 18. Nutritional Supplements

1. Paola Albertazzi. "Soy Supplement: Why Is the Effect So Elusive?" *The Journal of Clinical Endocrinology and Metabolism* 87, No. 7 (2002): 3508.

2. A. Singh, F.M. Moses, and P.A. Deuster. "Vitamin and Mineral Status in Physically Active Men: Effects of a High Potency Supplement." *American Journal of Clinical Nutrition* 55 (1992): 1–7.

Chapter 19. Integrative and Alternative Therapies

1. "The Use of Complementary and Alternative Medicine in the United States." National Center for Complementary and Alternative Medicine. Retrieved from http://nccam.nih.gov/news/camstats/2007/camsurvey_fs1.htm.

2. Stephen M. Kovel. *The International Academy of Oral Medicine and Toxicology* 9, (1995): 504–508. Retrieved from www.iaomt.org/articles/files/files/C3/the%20case%20against/%20amalgam.pdf

Chapter 20. Treating Minor Injuries and Illness

1. S.E. Efem. "Clinical Observations on the Wound Healing Properties of Honey." *Journal of Infection* 20, (July–August 1992): 227–229.

Resources

Throughout this book, I have recommended products that can help you live a healthier, more natural life. Some items, such as hydrogen peroxide, are easy to find in local stores. The following list was compiled to aid you in locating those items that can be a bit more difficult to find. As you will see, the companies are divided into categories such as "Air Purification," "Baby Care," "Bathroom Products," etc. For each firm, contact information, including website, is offered so that you can learn more about any products of interest, and order them if desired. Be aware that many of these firms carry more items than I have listed. I have included only those products with which I am familiar, and in which I have confidence. Don't feel that you must limit yourself to the resources shown below, though. New companies with great new products are cropping up all the time, so feel free to use your favorite search engine to find the natural, nontoxic items that will help you travel the road to health.

AIR PURIFICATION

American Air & Water, Inc.
12 Gibson Drive
Hilton Head Island, SC 29926
Phone: 888-378-4892
Toll Free: 888-378-4892
Fax: 843-785-2064
Website:
   www.americanairandwater.com
Email:
   sales@americanairandwater.com
This company offers ultraviolet air and water cleaners and purifiers that make your home environment safer.

Filters Fast, LLC
5905 Stockbridge Drive
Monroe, NC 28110
Phone: 866-438-3458
Website: www.filtersfast.com
Filters fast offers a 3M filtrete filter.

Gaiam
833 W. South Boulder Road
PO Box 3095
Boulder, CO 80307
Phone: 877-989-6321
Website: www.gaiam.com
Gaiam offers HEPA air purifiers and a window ventilator.

Second Wind
711 Park Avenue
Medina, NY 14103
Phone: 800-387-4565
Fax: 585-798-5751
Website:
  www.secondwindairpurifier.com
*Second Wind sells an air purification
system using ultraviolet light.*

BABY CARE

Baby Bunz & Company
PO Box 113
Lynden, WA 98264
Phone: 800-676-4559
Website: www.babybunz.com
Email: info@babybunz.com
*Baby Bunz offers a variety of natural baby
basics including blankets, diapers, diaper
cream, pajamas, and swim diapers.*

Born Free
2263 North West Boca Raton
  Boulevard, Suite 202
Boca Raton, FL 33431
Phone: 877-999-2676
Website: www.newbornfree.com
*Born Free sells bottle nipples, glass baby
bottles, pacifiers, plastic bottles, teethers,
and plastic training cups.*

Bumkins
7802 East Gray Road, Suite 500
Scottsdale, AZ 85260
Phone: 866-286-5467
Fax: 877-286-3511
Website: www.bumkins.com
*Bumkins offers natural, toxin-free baby
bibs, diapers, and tote bags.*

California Baby
5933 Bowcroft Street
Los Angeles, CA 90016
Phone: 310-815-8201
Website: www.californiababy.com
*California Baby offers a wide variety of
natural products including baby shampoo,
body wash, bubble bath, conditioner, diaper
cream, essential oil diffusers, hand soap,
lavender and lemon essential oils, and
mosquito repellent.*

Organic Comfort Zone
201 West Ocean View Avenue
Norfolk, VA 23503
Phone: 800-229-7571
Website:
  www.organiccomfortzone.com
Email: service@tomorrowsworld.com
*Organic Comfort Zone sells adult wool wet
pads, organic baby caps, cotton toys, kid
pillows, pajamas, and wool comforters.*

Seventh Generation
60 Lake Street
Burlington, VT 05401
Phone: 800-456-1191
Fax: 802-658-1771
Website: www.seventhgeneration.com
*Seventh Generation offers chlorine-free
diapers and wet wipes.*

BABY'S ROOM

DEX Products, Inc.
840 Eubanks Drive, Suite A
Vacaville, CA 95688
Phone: 800-546-1996
Website: www.dexbaby.com
Email: mail@dexproducts.com
*DEX offers a secure memory foam sleep
positioner that keeps baby in a safe position
all night.*

Life Kind
1415 Whispering Pines Lane, Suite 100
Grass Valley, CA 95945

Phone: 800-284-4983
Website: www.lifekind.com
Life Kind offers organic bedding, cribs, wool crib mattress, and wood furniture.

Nature Pedic
4370 Cranwood Parkway
Cleveland, OH 44128
Phone: 800-917-3342
Fax: 206-666-6613
Website: www.naturepedic.com
Nature Pedic sells certified organic blankets, crib mattresses, sheets, and wet pads, manufactured without harmful chemicals.

BATHROOM PRODUCTS

Bathroom Accessories Unlimited
1136-1146 Stratford Avenue
Stratford, CT 06615
Phone: 800-667-8721
Website: www.kitchensource.com/bau
Email: support@kitchensource.com
Bathroom Accessories Unlimited offers exhaust fans with timers, hampers, soap dishes, towel bars, towel rings, and soap dispensers.

Gaiam
833 West South Boulder Road
PO Box 3095
Boulder, CO 80307
Phone: 877-989-6321
Website: www.gaiam.com
Gaiam offers linen shower curtains.

Green Nest
18662 MacArthur Boulevard, Suite 200
Irvine, CA 92612
Phone: 888-473-6466
Website: www.greennest.com
Email: support@greennest.com
Green Nest sells organic shower curtains.

Hair Doc
9136 Desoto Avenue
Chatsworth, CA 91311
Phone: 818-882-4247
Website: www.thehairdoccompany.com
The Hair Doc Company offers combs, hair brushes, loofah gloves, razors, shaving brushes, and toothbrushes.

Rawganique.com
Phone: 877-729-4367
Website: www.rawganique.com
Rawganique offers organic hemp shower curtains.

BEDROOM PRODUCTS

Advanced Sleep Products
8191 Roosevelt Avenue
Midway City, CA 92655
Phone: 800-877-5337
Fax: 714-890-1426
Website: www.advancedsleepproducts.com
Email: info@advancedsleepproducts.com
Advanced Sleep Products offers air, foam, and water mattresses; bed foundations; and bed frames.

Clean Brands, LLC
400 Massassoit Avenue, Suite 300
East Providence, RI 02914
Phone: 877-215-7378
Fax: 401-437-8483
Website: www.cleanrest.com
Email: info@cleanrest.com
Clean Brands offers dust mite-proof bed and pillow coverings.

Gaiam
833 West South Boulder Road
PO Box 3095

Boulder, CO 80307
Phone: 877-989-6321
Website: www.gaiam.com
Gaiam offers organic bed linens and
natural alarm lights.

Green Nest
18662 MacArthur Boulevard Suite 200
Irvine, CA 92612
Phone: 888-473-6466
Website: www.greennest.com
Email: support@greennest.com
Green Nest offers organic bed linens.

Promo Life
3656 Dead Horse Mountain Road
Fayetteville, AR 72701
Phone: 888-742-3404
Fax: 479-444-6422
Website: www.promolife.com
Promo Life offers magnetic mattress pads.

Tempur-Pedic
1713 Jaggie Fox Way
Lexington, KY 40511
Phone: 888-811-5053
Website: www.tempurpedic.com
Email: drsupportemail@
   tempurpedicdr.com
Tempur-Pedic sells bed frames, bed linens,
foam mattresses, foam pillows, and
foundations.

CAR CARE

BeFreeTech.com
285 West Country Circle Drive
Port Orange, FL 32128
Phone: 386-868-2846
Website: www.befreetech.com
Email: store@befreetech.com
BeFreeTech.com offers 100-percent
natural hydrocarbon refrigerants,
a healthful alternative to freon.

Laura Klein's Green Cleaning
9190 West Olympia Boulevard, Suite
   305
Beverly Hills, CA 90212
Phone: 310-694-8306
Fax: 310-388-0357
Website:
   www.laurakleinsgreencleaning.com
Email:
   info@laurakleinsgreencleaning.com
Laura Klein's Green Cleaning offers
nontoxic exterior car cleaners and
protectors.

CLOTHING

Gaiam
833 West South Boulder Road
PO Box 3095
Boulder, CO 80307
Phone: 877-989-6321
Website: www.gaiam.com
Gaiam offers natural footwear and organic
undergarments, robes, sleepwear, and
towels.

Maggie's Functional Organics
306 West Cross Street
Ypsilanti, MI 48197
Phone: 800-609-8593
Fax: 734-482-4175
Website: www.maggiesorganics.com
Email: maggies@organicclothes.com
Maggie's Functional Organics offers
camisoles, halter tops, loungewear, pants,
shirts, socks, and tights.

COOKWARE

Barbecuewood.com
PO Box 8163
Yakima, WA 98908
Phone: 800-379-9663
Website: www.barbecuewood.com

Email: sales@bbqwoods.com
Barbecuewood.com sells electric grills.

CorningWare
1200 South Antrim Way
Greencastle, PA 17225
Phone: 800-999-3436
Website: www.corningware.com
Email: helpcenter@worldkitchen.com
*CorningWare offers ceramic and glass
cookware.*

Gaiam
833 West South Boulder Road
PO Box 3095
Boulder, CO 80307
Phone: 877-989-6321
Website: www.gaiam.com
Gaiam sells a convection oven.

The Pampered Chef
One Pampered Chef Lane
Addison, IL 60101
Phone: 888-687-2433
Website: www.pamperedchef.com
The Pampered Chef offers stone bakeware.

EMF PROTECTION

Cutting Edge
PO Box 4158
Santa Fe, NM 87502
Phone: 800-497-9516
Website: www.cutcat.com
Email: cutcat@cutcat.com
*Cutting Edge offers Gauss meter EMF
meters, EMF and geopathic stress
protection products, and photoelectric
smoke detectors.*

Ener-G-Polari-T
PO Box 12430
Scottsdale, AZ 85267
Phone: 800-593-6374

Website: www.energpolarit.com
Email: info@energpolarit.com
*Ener-G-Polari-T offers cell phone and
cordless phone diodes, circuit breaker
diodes, and computer diodes.*

EXERCISE EQUIPMENT

Endless Pools
1601 Dutton Mill Road
Aston, PA 19014
Phone: 800-732-8660
Fax: 610-497-9328
Website: www.endlesspools.com
Email: swim@endlesspools.com
*Endless Pools sells the Fastlane Pool and
in-home swimming pools.*

FitMed
PO Box 183
Mill Valley, CA 94942
Phone: 800-959-4089
Website: www.heartmonitors.com
Email: support@heartmonitors.com
FitMed sells heart rate monitors.

Gaiam
833 West South Boulder Road
PO Box 3095
Boulder, CO 80307
Phone: 877-989-6321
Website: www.gaiam.com
*Gaiam offers body slant cushions and
pinhole eyeglasses.*

Kiefer
1700 Kiefer Drive
Zion, IL 60099
Phone: 800-323-4071
Fax: 800-654-7946
Website: www.kiefer.com
Email: info@kiefer.com
*Kiefer sells an aqua jogger flotation vest,
foam exercise equipment, and pool shoes.*

Needak Manufacturing
120 West Douglas Street
O'Neill, NE 68763
Phone: 800-232-5762
Website: www.needakrebounders.com
*Needak offers hand weights and
rebounders.*

New Balance
Brighton Landing
20 Guest Street
Boston, MA 02135
Phone: 800-253-7463
Website: www.newbalance.com
*New Balance sells running and walking
shoes.*

Selle SMP
Via Einstein, 5
35020 Casalserugo, Italy
Phone: +39-049-643966
Website: www.sellesmp.com
Email: info@sellesmp.com
*Selle SMP offers an open-cut bicycle
seat.*

Ski Walking
5873 Lake Street
PO Box 322
Glen Arbor, MI 49636
Phone: 877-754-9255
Website: www.skiwalking.com
Email: getfit@skiwalking.com
*Ski Walking sells Nordic Ski Walking
poles.*

Teeter Hang Ups
9902 162nd Street Court East
Puyallup, WA 98375
Phone: 800-718-1710
Fax: 800-847-0188
Website: www.teeter-inversion.com
*Teeter Hang Ups sells an inversion
board.*

True Fitness
865 Hoff Road
St. Louis, MO 63366
Phone: 800-426-6570
Website: www.truefitness.com
Email: info@truefitness.com
True sells treadmills.

FOOD AND COSMETIC CONTAINERS

Container & Packaging Supply
1345 East State Street
Eagle, ID 83616
Phone: 800-473-4144
Website:
   www.containerandpackaging.com
*Container & Packaging Supply offers
cosmetic tubes, caps, pumps, glass bottles
for cosmetic storage, glass containers for
food, and travel-size containers.*

Crate and Barrel
Phone: 800-967-6696
Website: www.crateandbarrel.com
*Crate and Barrel offers glass containers for
food. Visit their website for the nearest store.*

FOOD PRODUCTS

BABY FOOD

Earth's Best
4600 Sleepytime Drive
Boulder, CO 80301
Phone: 800-434-4246
Website: www.earthsbest.com
*Earth's Best offers organic cereal, fruit, and
vegetables. Their products are available in
many natural food stores and online.*

Gerber Baby
445 State Street
Freemont, MI 49413
Phone: 800-443-7237

Website: www.gerber.com

Gerber offers organic cereal, fruit, and vegetables.

BEVERAGES

Diamond Organics
1272 Highway 1
Moss Landing, CA 95039
Phone: 888-674-2642
Website: www.diamondorganics.com
Email: info@diamondorganics.com

Diamond Organics offers organic alcoholic and nonalcoholic beverages, decaffeinated coffee, juice, and tea.

BREADS AND PASTA

Diamond Organics
1272 Highway 1
Moss Landing, CA 95039
Phone: 888-674-2642
Website: www.diamondorganics.com

Diamond Organics offers organic lasagna, linguine, penne, ravioli, and spaghetti.

Rudi's Organic Bakery
3300 Walnut Street, Unit C
Boulder, CO 80301
Phone: 877-293-0876
Website: www.rudisbakery.com

Rudi's Organic Bakery offers organic bagels, buns, muffins, rolls, tortilla wraps, and a variety of breads. Look on their website for the retailer nearest you.

CONDIMENTS

Arrowhead Mills
4600 Sleepytime Drive
Boulder, CO 80301
Phone: 800-434-4246
Website: www.arrowheadmills.com

Arrowhead Mills sells quality almond butter and peanut butter.

Diamond Organics
1272 Highway 1
Moss Landing, CA 95039
Phone: 888-674-2642
Website: www.diamondorganics.com

Diamond Organics offers coconut oil, flax oil, jams, ketchup, olive oil, sea salt, and syrup.

Eden Organic
701 Tecumseh Road
Clinton, MI 49236
Phone: 888-424-3336
Website: www.edenfoods.com
Email: info@edenfoods.com

Eden sells raw apple cider vinegar.

Nutiva
PO Box 1716
Sebastopol, CA 95473
Phone: 800-993-4367
Website: www.nutiva.com
Email: help1@nutiva.com

Nutiva offers coconut oil.

Spectrum
4600 Sleepytime Drive
Boulder, CO 80301
Phone: 800-434-4246
Website: www.spectrumorganics.com
Email:
    spectrumorganics@worldpantry.com

Spectrum offers coconut oil, flax oil, olive oil, and raw apple cider vinegar.

DAIRY ALTERNATIVES

Blue Diamond
PO Box 1768
Sacramento, CA 95812
Phone: 800-987-2329
Website: www.bluediamond.com

Blue Diamond offers Almond Breeze, an almond milk product. Their products are available online and in many supermarkets.

Dairy Products

Anala Goat Company
15501 Alton Road
Beasley, TX 77417
Phone: 281-343-5991
Website: www.analagoatcompany.com
Email:
    mother@analagoatcompany.com
The Anala Goat Company offers eggs, goat cheese, goat's milk, and kefir.

Diamond Organics
1272 Highway 1
Moss Landing, CA 95039
Phone: 888-674-2642
Website: www.diamondorganics.com
Diamond Organics offers organic butter, eggs, goat cheese, and yogurt.

Laloo's
Phone: 707-763-1491
Website: www.laloos.com
Email: laloo@laloos.com
Laloo's offers goat's milk ice cream and goat's milk frozen yogurt. Their products may be ordered online or found in your local Whole Foods Market and other health food stores.

Meyenberg
PO Box 934
Turlock, CA 95381
Phone: 800-891-4628
Fax: 209-668-4977
Website: www.meyenberg.com
Email: info@meyenberg.com
Meyenberg produces goat butter, goat cheese, and goat's milk.

Organic Valley
CROPP Cooperative
One Organic Way
LaFarge, WI 54639
Phone: 888-444-6455
Fax: 608-625-3025
Website: www.organicvalley.coop
Organic Valley offers organic butter, cheese, eggs, and raw milk.

Tree of Life
405 Golfway West Drive
St. Augustine, FL 32095
Phone: 904-940-2100
Fax: 904-940-2264
Website: www.treeeoflife.com
Email: mailbox@treeoflife.com
Tree of Life offers organic cheese, eggs, and raw milk.

Desserts and Snacks

Back to Nature
PO Box 8995
Madison, WI 53708
Phone: 866-536-6946
Website: www.backtonaturefoods.com
Back to Nature sells natural cookies, crackers, granolas, roasted and unroasted nuts, and trail mix.

Diamond Organics
1272 Highway 1
Moss Landing, CA 95039
Phone: 888-674-2642
Website: www.diamondorganics.com
Diamond Organics offers organic candies, health bars, and trail mix.

Fruits and Vegetables

Diamond Organics
1272 Highway 1
Moss Landing, CA 95039
Phone: 888-674-2642
Website: www.diamondorganics.com
Diamond Organics offers a large assortment of organic fruits and vegetables.

Whole Foods Market, Inc.
550 Bowie Street
Austin, TX 78703
Phone: 512-477-4455
Fax: 512-482-7000
Website: www.wholefoodsmarket.com
Email: customer.questions@
wholefoods.com

Whole Foods Market offers a large assortment of fruits and vegetables. Visit their website to find a store nearest you.

GRAINS, NUTS, SEEDS, AND LEGUMES

Arrowhead Mills
4600 Sleepytime Drive
Boulder, CO 80301
Phone: 800-749-0730
Website: www.arrowheadmills.com

Arrowhead Mills offers cooking mixes, gluten-free products, grains, legumes, and seeds.

Bob's Red Mill
13521 South East Pheasant Court
Milwaukie, OR 97222
Phone: 800-349-2173
Fax: 503-653-1339
Website: www.bobsredmill.com

Bob's Red Mill offers aluminum-free baking soda, cereals, gluten-free products, grains, and legumes. Their products are found in many local supermarkets and can be ordered from their website.

MEAT, POULTRY, AND SEAFOOD

Diamond Organics
1272 Highway 1
Moss Landing, CA 95039
Phone: 888-674-2642
Website: www.diamondorganics.com

Diamond Organics offers organic beef, lamb, and poultry; grass-fed buffalo; and wild seafood.

EcoFish, Inc.
340 Central Ave.
Dover, NH 03820
Phone: 877-214-3474
Website: www.ecofish.com
Email: comments@ecofish.com

EcoFish offers a variety of wild seafood.

Maverick Ranch
5320 North Franklin Street
Denver, CO 80216
Phone: 303-294-0026
Website: www.maverickranch.com
Email: info@maverickranch.com

Maverick Ranch offers organic beef, natural buffalo, and free-range lamb and poultry.

White Egret Farm
15704 Webberville Road
FM 969
Austin, TX 78724
Phone: 512-300-3584
Fax: 512-276-7489
Website: www.whiteegretfarm.com

White Egret Farm offers natural beef and free-range poultry.

SWEETENERS

Diamond Organics
1272 Highway 1
Moss Landing, CA 95039
Phone: 888-674-2642
Website: www.diamondorganics.com

Diamond Organics offers organic powdered sugar and Turbinado sugar.

Walker Farms
6251 Bee Charmer Lane
North Fort Myers, FL 33917
Phone: 239-543-8071
Fax: 239-543-8762
Website: www.walkerfarmshoney.com
Email: info@walkerfarmshoney.com

Walker Farms sells raw honey.

Wholesome Sweeteners, Inc.
8016 Highway 90-A
Sugar Land, TX 77478
Phone: 800-680-1896
Fax: 281-275-3170
Website: www.organicsugars.biz
Email: CS@organicsugar.biz
Wholesome Sweeteners offers brown sugar, molasses, Sucanat, and Turbinado sugar.

FOOD STORAGE

Gaiam
833 West South Boulder Road
PO Box 3095
Boulder, CO 80307
Phone: 877-989-6321
Canada: 800-254-8464
Website: www.gaiam.com
Gaiam offers vacuum food storage containers.

Natural Value
14 Waterthrush Court
Sacramento, CA 95831
Phone: 916-427-7242
Fax: 916-427-3784
Website: www.naturalvalue.com
Email: info@naturalvalue.com
Natural Value offers biodegradable garbage bags, plastic storage bags, and unbleached waxed paper.

HAIR AND MAKEUP

Ecco Bella
623 Eagle Rock Road, Suite 381
Montclair, NJ 07042
Phone: 877-696-2220
Website: www.eccobella.com
Email:
    customer_service@eccobella.com
Ecco Bella offers natural blush, concealer,

eyeliner, eye shadow, foundation, lipstick, and hair-care products.

Giovanni
PO Box 6990
Beverly Hills, CA 90212
Phone: 310-952-9960
Website: www.giovannicosmetics.com
Email: info@giovannicosmetics.com
Giovanni offers organic hair gel and hair sprays.

Light Mountain Natural
PO Box 325
Twin Lakes, WI 53181
Phone: 262-889-8561
Fax: 262-889-2461
Website: www.light-mountain-hair-
    color.com
Email: lightmountain@lotuspress.com
Light Mountain Natural offers herbal hair coloring.

Sears
Phone: 1-800-349-4358
Website: www.sears.com
Sears offers asbestos-free hair dryers, which include all Conair and Remington models. Call or go online to find the store that's nearest you.

HEALTH AND NUTRITIONAL SUPPORT

CC Pollen Company
3627 East Indian School Road, Suite 209
Phoenix, AZ 85018
Phone: 800-875-0096
Website: www.ccpollen.com
Email: response@ccpollen.com
CC Pollen Company offers bee pollen, propolis, and royal jelly.

Internatural
PO Box 489
Twin Lakes, WI 53181
Phone: 800-643-4221
Fax: 800-905-6887
Website: www.internatural.com
Email:
   customersupport@internatural.com
Internatural offers Neti Pots.

Lily of the Desert
1887 Geesling Road
Denton, TX 76208
Phone: 800-229-5459
Website: www.lilyofthedesert.com
Lily of the Desert offers aloe vera juice.

Natren
3105 Willow Lane
West Lake Village, CA 91361
Phone: 866-462-8736
Website: www.natren.com
Natren sells probiotics in a goat milk base.

The Synergy Company
2279 South Resource Boulevard
Moab, UT 84532
Phone: 800-723-0277
Fax: 435-259-2328
Website:
   www.thesynergycompany.com
Email: customer-service@synergy-
   co.com
*The Synergy Company offers Pure
Synergy, an organic superfood, and blue-
green algae.*

Tao of Herbs, Inc.
3340 South Wallace Street
Chicago, IL 60616
Phone: 312-881-0078
Website: www.taoofherbs.com
Email: info@taoofherbs.com

*Tao of Herbs sells peppermint essential oil
and red raspberry leaf tea.*

HOME FURNISHINGS

Earth Shade
PO Box 1003
Barrington, MA 01230
Phone: 413-528-5443
Website: www.earthshade.com
Email: info@earthshade.com
*Earth Shade offers natural window
coverings.*

Eco Haus
4121 First Avenue South
Seattle, WA 98134
Phone: 877-432-6428
Website: www.ecohaus.com
*Eco Haus offers wood furniture and other
green home furnishings. Visit the website
to see if there's a dealer near you.*

Furnature
86 Coolidge Avenue
Watertown, MA 02472
Phone: 800-326-4895
Website: www.furnature.com
*Furnature offers cotton foam furniture,
cotton and hemp fabrics, and pillows.*

Gaiam
833 West South Boulder Road
PO Box 3095
Boulder, CO 80307
Phone: 877-989-6321
Website: www.gaiam.com
*Gaiam offers full-spectrum lighting as well
as furniture coverings.*

Mod Green Pod
1507 West Koenig Lane
Austin, TX 78756

Phone: 512-524-5196
Fax: 610-602-2765
Website: www.modgreenpod.com
Email: info@modgreenpod.com
Mod Green Pod supplies organic fabric and wallpaper.

Natural Area Rugs
8306 Wilshire Boulevard, Suite 4500
Beverly Hills, CA 90211
Phone: 800-661-7847
Fax: 323-582-1117
Website: www.naturalarearugs.com
Email: info@naturalarearugs.com
Natural Area Rugs offers flooring made of natural fibers such as bamboo and seagrass.

Naturlich
7120 Keating Avenue
Sebastopol, CA 95472
Phone: 707-829-3959
Fax: 707-829-1774
Website: www.naturalfloors.net
Email: info@naturalfloors.net
Naturlich sells natural draperies, natural shades and other window treatments, and natural flooring.

HOME IMPROVEMENT

Bryant
Phone: 800-428-4326
Website: www.bryant.com
Bryant manufactures custom air filters, cooling and heating systems, thermostats, and thermidistats. Call or visit their website to find a dealer near you.

Eco Haus
4121 First Avenue South
Seattle, WA 98134
Phone: 877-432-6428
Website: www.ecohaus.com
Eco Haus offers natural, nontoxic

adhesives, cabinets, caulking, cotton insulation, countertops, decks, grout, hardwood flooring, wool carpeting, linoleum, paints, primers, and sealers. Call or visit the website to see if there's a dealer near you.

Green Building Supply
508 North 2nd Street
Fairfield, IA 52556
Phone: 800-405-0222
Website:
   www.greenbuildingsupply.com
Email:
   info1@greenbuildingsupply.com
Green Building Supply sells natural, nontoxic adhesives, carpet, carpet pads, caulking, cement, glue, grout, paint remover, hardwood and plywood sealers, stain, stucco sealers, and tile.

Green Nest
18662 MacArthur Boulevard, Suite 200
Irvine, CA 92612
Phone: 888-473-6466
Website: www.greennest.com
Email: support@greennest.com
Green Nest offers nontoxic carpet sealer, carpet shampoo, mold prevention sealer, paints, and primers.

The Home Depot
Phone: 800-553-3199
Website: www.homedepot.com
The Home Depot offers carbon monoxide detectors, face masks, and solar panels. Call or visit their website to find the store nearest you.

HOME PEST CONTROL

Orange Guard
Phone: 888-659-3217
Fax: 831-659-5128

Website: www.orangeguard.com
Email: orangeguard@sbcglobal.net
Orange Guard offers a natural insect spray repellent. This product can be found at your local Whole Foods Market or ACE Hardware store, or ordered online.

Smart Home
16542 Millikan Avenue
Irvine, CA 92606
Phone: 800-762-7846
Fax: 800-242-7329
Website: www.smarthome.com
Email: custsvc@smarthome.com
Smart Home sells a sonic rodent deterrent.

HOUSEHOLD CLEANERS

Brushtech
4 Matt Avenue
PO Box 1130
Plattsburgh, NY 12901
Phone: 518-563-2401
Fax: 518-563-0581
Website: www.brushtechbrushes.com
Brushtech sells bathroom brushes, dryer vent brushes, kitchen brushes, and toilet brushes.

Citra Solv
PO Box 2597
Danbury, CT 06813
Phone: 800-343-6588
Website: www.citra-solv.com
Email: info@citrasolv.com
Citra Solv offers natural dishwashing soap, drain cleaner, glass cleaner, laundry detergent, and window cleaner.

Dr. Bronner's Magic Soaps
PO Box 28
Escondido, CA 92033
Phone: 760-743-2211
Website: www.drbronner.com

Dr. Bronner's offers natural all-purpose hard surface and tile cleaners, as well as peppermint soap.

Eco Discoveries
2377 John Glenn Drive Suite 106
Atlanta, GA 30341
Phone: 866-767-2832
Website: www.ecodiscoveries.com
Email: smoore@ecodiscoveries.com
Eco Discoveries offers natural nursery cleaner, Moldzyme mold remover, Multizyme all-purpose cleaner, and tile cleaner.

Seventh Generation
60 Lake Street
Burlington, VT 05401
Phone: 800-456-1191
Fax: 802-658-1771
Website: www.seventhgeneration.com
Seventh Generation offers chlorine-free bleach and safe, environmentally responsible laundry detergent, napkins, paper towels, tissues, and toilet paper.

INSPIRATIONAL MATERIALS

Guideposts
PO Box 5814
Harlan, IA 51593
Phone: 800-431-2344
Website: www.guideposts.com
Guideposts is a magazine featuring inspiring people stories.

Insight for Living
PO Box 269000
Plano, TX 75026
Phone: 800-772-8888
Website: www.insight.org
Insight for Living provides a Christian radio broadcast and inspirational literature.

KITCHEN PRODUCTS

Eco Wise
110 West Elizabeth
Austin, TX 78704
Phone: 512-326-4474
Fax: 512-326-4496
Website: www.ecowise.com
Eco Wise sells beeswax candles and chlorine-free paper cups and plates.

If You Care
Phone: 201-947-1000
Website: www.ifyoucare.com
Email:
   ifyoucare@foodimportgroup.com
If You Care offers all natural waxed paper, chlorine-free coffee filters, and parchment baking paper. Their products can be found in your Whole Foods Market or online.

Gourmet Depot
840 Folsom Street
San Francisco, CA 94107
Phone: 800-424-6783
Website: www.thegourmetdepot.net
Gourmet Depot offers blenders and bread makers.

Tristar Products, Inc.
PO Box 3007
Wallingford, CT 06492
Phone: 973-287-5150
Website: www.powerjuicer.com
Tristar Products, Inc. sells the Jack LaLanne Power Juicer. You can order it online or find it in your local Target store.

LAWN AND GARDEN CARE

Arbico Organics
PO Box 8910
Tucson, AZ 85738
Phone: 800-827-2847
Website: www.arbico-organics.com
Email: service@arbico.com
Arbico Organics offers organic garden and lawn fertilizer, natural weed and disease control products, and insecticides.

Garden Guys
Phone: 888-473-6489
         508-823-1117
Website: www.garden-guys.com
Email: info@garden-guys.com
Garden Guys offers natural fertilizer and neem oil-based garden bug repellent.

Planet Natural
1612 Gold Avenue.
Bozeman, MT 59715
Phone: 406-587-5891
Fax: 406-587-0223
Website: www.planetnatural.com
Planet Natural sells corn-gluten meal, organic fertilizer, natural insecticides, and lawnmowers.

ORAL CARE

Eco Dent
PO Box 489
Twin Lakes, WI 53181
Phone: 877-263-9456
Fax: 262-889-8591
Website: www.eco-dent.com
Eco-Dent offers natural mouthwash, fluoride-free toothpaste, and unwaxed dental floss.

Hydro Floss
3030 Dublin Circle
Bessemer, AL 35022
Phone: 800-635-3594
Fax: 888-258-4504
Website: www.hydrofloss.com
Email: helpdesk@hydrofloss.com
Hydro Floss sells oral irrigators.

Jason Natural Cosmetics
PO Box 5058
Gardena, CA 90249
Phone: 877-538-3553
Website: www.jasoncosmetics.com
Jason Cosmetics sells natural mouthwash and toothpaste.

PERSONAL CARE

Aubrey Organics
4419 North Manhatten Avenue
Tampa, FL 33614
Phone: 800-282-7394
Fax: 813-876-8166
Website: www.aubrey-organics.com
Aubrey Organics offers natural aftershave, deodorant, lip balm, and shaving cream.

Burt's Bees
PO Box 13489
Durham, NC 27709
Phone: 800-849-7112
Website: www.burtsbees.com
Burt's Bees offers natural body lotion, body wash, conditioner, lip balm, shampoo, and sunscreen.

CC Pollen Company
3627 East Indian School Road, Suite 209
Phoenix, AZ 85018
Phone: 800-875-0096
Website: www.ccpollen.com
Email: response@ccpollen.com
CC Pollen offers natural face creams and face masks.

Clear Conscience
PO Box 17855
Arlington, VA 22216
Phone: 800-595-9592
Website: www.clearconscience.com
Email: info@clearconscience.com

Clear Conscience offers safe contact lens cases and solutions.

Desert Essence
PO Box 14007
Hauppauge, NY 11788
Website: www.desertessence.com
Email:
    customercare@desertessence.com
Desert Essence sells coconut hand and body lotion, conditioner, jojoba oil, and shampoo.

Dr. Bronner's Magic Soaps
PO Box 28
Escondido, CA 92033
Phone: 760-743-2211
Fax: 760-745-6675
Website: www.drbronner.com
Dr. Bronner's offers organic shaving gel and soap.

Honey Bee Gardens
200 Penn Avenue
West Reading, PA 19611
Phone: 610-396-9225
Website: www.honeybeegardens.com
Email: sales@honeybeegardens.com
Honey Bee Gardens sells natural facial toners and cosmetics, toxin-free odorless nail polish and remover, nail file buffers, and pedicure kits.

Internatural
PO Box 489
Twin Lakes, WI 53181
Phone: 800-643-4221
Fax: 800-905-6887
Website: www.internatural.com
Email:
    customersupport@internatural.com
Internatural offers natural men's cologne and shaving cream.

Kiss My Face
PO Box 224
1144 Main Street
Gardiner, NY 12525
Phone: 800-262-5477
Fax: 845-255-4312
Website: www.kissmyface.com
Kiss My Face sells natural hand and body soaps.

Lice B Gone
PO Box 528
Belleville, IL 62222
Phone: 877-730-2727
Fax: 618-236-2826
Website: www.licebgone.com
Lice B Gone offers natural shampoos for lice, nits, and scabies.

Tiger Flag Natural Perfumery
6040 East Main Street Suite 190
Mesa, AZ 85205
Phone: 480-833-4562
Website: www.tigerflag.com
Email: perfumeinfo@tigerflag.com
Tiger Flag Natural Perfumery offers natural and organic women's perfume.

Seventh Generation
60 Lake Street
Burlington, VT 05401
Phone: 800-456-1191
Fax: 802-658-1771
Website: www.seventhgeneration.com
Seventh Generation offers chlorine-free, organic feminine hygiene products.

PET CARE

All Green Things
5321 Topanga Canyon Boulevard
Woodland Hills, CA 91364
Phone: 877-326-7763
Fax: 818-716-7544

Website: www.allgreenthings.com
Email: info@allgreenthings.com
All Green Things sells conditioner, dog beds, grooming wipes, hemp collars, hemp leashes, natural shampoo, toys, and waste bags.

Local Harvest
220 21st Avenue
Santa Cruz, CA 95062
Phone: 831-515-5602
Website: www.localharvest.org
Local harvest offers safe flea collars and toys, and organic pet food.

Smart Home
16542 Millikan Avenue
Irvine, CA 92606
Phone: 800-762-7846
Fax: 800-242-7329
Website: www.smarthome.com
Email: custsvc@smarthome.com
Smart Home sells electronic yard fences.

PREGNANCY AND NURSING

Baby Nut
1403 19th Street
Bellingham, WA 98225
Phone: 800-671-3679
Website: www.babynut.com
Email: help@babynut.com
Baby Nut sells organic baby clothes, books, maternity clothes, nursing clothes, music, and toys.

Medela
1101 Corporate Drive
McHenry, IL 60050
Phone: 800-435-8316
Fax: 815-363-1246
Website: www.medela.com
Medela offers breast milk storage bags and bottles, breast pumps, and nursing pads.

Nature's Crib
201 CR 31
Glen Spey, NY 12737
Phone: 845-313-2371
845-856-9042
Website: www.naturescrib.com
Email: support@naturescrib.com
Nature's Crib offers organic baby bedding,
baby carriers, baby clothes, breast creams,
nursing pillows, and toys.

REED DIFFUSERS

V.I. Reed and Crane Inc.
8522 Lakeview Bay Road
Rogers, AR 72756
Phone: 800-852-0025
Fax: 561-828-5968
Website: www.reeddiffusers.org
Email: info@reeddiffusers.org
V.I. Reed and Crane offers products for reed
diffusers, including bottles, reeds, and
essential oils.

SAUNAS

Fauna Sauna
Wavemaker LLC
2721 Shattuck Avenue, Suite 224
Berkeley, CA 94705
Phone: 877-732-5196
Fax: 510-740-3971
Website: www.faunasauna.com
Fauna Sauna sells far infrared radiant
heaters and heated furniture for pets.

Sunlighten
7373 West 107th Street
Overland Park, KS 66212
Phone: 913-754-0831
Website: www.sunlighten.com
Email: info@sunlightsaunas.com
Sunlighten offers far infrared saunas.

SWIMMING POOL AND SPA SANITATION

Del Ozone
3580 Sueldo Street
San Luis Obispo, CA 93401
Phone: 800-676-1335
Website: www.delzone.com
Email: residentialpools@delzone.com
Del Ozone offers water purification
systems using ozone.

Ecosmarte Pool
Phone: 866-246-3546
Website: www.ecosmartepool.com
Ecosmarte Pool offers water purification
using ionization.

Nature²
2620 Commerce Way
Vista, CA 92081
Phone: 800-822-7933
Website: www.nature2.com
Email: sales@zpc.zodiac.com
Nature² offers water purification systems
using minerals.

VACUUM CLEANERS

Goodman's
10914 NW 33rd Street, Suite 107
Miami, FL 33172
Phone: 888-333-4660
Fax: 305-278-1888
Website: www.goodmans.net
Goodman's offers steam cleaners.

Green Nest
18662 MacArthur Boulevard, Suite 200
Irvine, CA 92612
Phone: 888-473-6466
Website: www.greennest.com
Email: support@greennest.com
Green Nest offers HEPA vacuum cleaners.

WATER

Enviro Products
PO Box 4146
Englewood, CO 80155
Phone: 800-592-8371
Website: www.newwaveenviro.com
Enviro Products offers bathtub filters and reverse osmosis water filtration systems.

Gaiam
833 West South Boulder Road
PO Box 3095
Boulder, CO 80307
Phone: 877-989-6321
Website: www.gaiam.com
Gaiam offers polycarbonate bottles, reverse osmosis water filtration systems, and whole house filter systems.

Water Wise
3608 Parkway Boulevard
Leesburg, FL 34748
Phone: 800-874-9028
Fax: 866-329-8123
Website: www.waterwise.com
Email: sales@waterwise.com
Water Wise offers shower filters and water distillers.

Suggested Reading List

Anderson, Nina, and Howard Peiper. *Are You Poisoning Your Pets? A Guidebook to How Our Lifestyles Affect the Health of Our Pets.* Garden City Park, NY: Avery Publishing Group, 1998.

Banik, Allen E. *The Choice Is Clear.* Austin, TX: Acres USA, 1997.

Bates, W.H. *The Cure of Imperfect Sight by Treatment Without Glasses.* Pomeroy, WA: Health Research Books, 1920.

Becker, O. Robert, and Gary Sheldon. *The Body Electric: Electromagnetism and the Foundation of Life.* New York; William Morrow and Company Inc., 1998.

Benz, Reinhold. *Facebuilding: The Daily 5-Minute Program for a Beautiful, Wrinkle-Free Face.* New York: Sterling Publishing Company, 1991.

Berkson, Lindsey. *Hormone Deception: How Everyday Foods and Products Are Disrupting Your Hormones—and How to Protect Yourself and Your Family.* New York: McGraw-Hill, 2001.

Blaylock, Russell. *Excitotoxins: The Taste That Kills.* Santa Fe, NM: Health Press, 1996.

Bond-Berthold, Annie. *Better Basics for the Home.* New York: Tree Rivers Press, 1999.

Brown, Royden. *Bee Hive Product Bible.* Garden City Park, NY: Avery Publishing Group, 1993.

Campbell, Don. *The Mozart Effect: Tapping the Power of Music to Heal the Body, Strengthen the Mind, and Unlock the Creative Spirit.* New York: Avon Books Inc., 1997.

Carson, Rachel. *Silent Spring.* Boston: Houghton Mifflin, 1962.

Denckla, Tanya. *The Gardener's A-Z Guide to Growing Organic Food.* North Adams, MA: Storey Publishing LLC., 2003.

Fife, Bruce, and Jon J. Kabara. *The Coconut Oil Miracle.* Fourth Edition. New York: Penguin Group, 2004.

Frazine, Richard. *The Barefoot Hiker: A Book About Bare Feet and How Their Sensitivity Can Provide Not Only a Unique Dimension of Pleasure, but Also Significant Benefits.* Berkeley, CA: Ten Speed Press, 1993.

Goldberg, Gerald. *Would You Put Your Head in a Microwave Oven?* Bloomington, IN: Author House, 2006.

Groves, Barry. *Fluoride: Drinking Ourselves to Death*. Lithia Springs, GA: New Leaf Distributing Company, 2002.

Hobday, Richard. *The Healing Sun: Sunlight and Health in the 21st Century*. Forres, Scotland: Find Horn Press Ltd., 2000.

Jensen, Bernard, and Mark Anderson. *Empty Harvest*. New York: Penguin Group, 1995.

Jerome, Frank. *Tooth Truth*. Chula Vista, CA: New Century Press, 2000.

Lacey, Louise. *Lunaception: A Feminine Odyssey Into Fertility and Contraception*. New York: Coward, McCann and Geoghegan Inc., 1975.

Lopez, Andrew. *Natural Pest Control: Alternatives to Chemicals for the Home and Garden*. Fifteenth Edition. Malibu, CA: Invisible Gardener, 2008.

Maffetone, Philip. *Fix Your Feet: Build the Best Foundation for Healthy, Pain-Free Knees, Hips, and Spine*. Guilford, CT: Lyons Press, 2003.

Meyerowitz, Steve. *Power Juices, Super Drinks: Quick, Delicious Recipes to Prevent and Reverse Disease*. New York: Kensington Publishing, 2000.

Miller, Neil. *Vaccines: Are They Really Safe and Effective?* Santa Fe, NM: New Atlantean Press, 2008.

Mongan, Marie F. *HypnoBirthing: The Mongan Method*. Third Edition. Deerfield Beach, FL: Health Communications Inc., 2005.

Peale, Norman Vincent. *The Power of Positive Thinking*. New York: Ballantine Books, 1996.

Pinsky, Mark. *EMF Book: What You Should Know About Electromagnetic Fields*. Boston: Grand Central Publishing, 1995.

Sears, Martha, and William Sears. *The Breastfeeding Book: Everything You Need to Know About Nursing Your Child*. New York: Little, Brown and Company, 2000.

Statham, Bill. *The Chemical Maze Shopping Companion: Your Guide to Food Additives and Cosmetic Ingredients*. Second Edition. Adelaide, South Australia: Possibility.Com, 2005.

Sydney, Ross Singer, and Soma Grismaijer. *Dressed to Kill: The Link Between Breast Cancer and Bras*. Garden City Park, NY: Avery Publishing Group, 1995.

Thompson, Athena. *Homes That Heal (and those that don't): How Your Home Could be Harming Your Family's Health*. Gabriola Island, BC: New Society Publishers, 2004.

Walker, Norman W. *Colon Health: The Key to a Vibrant Life*. Boise, ID: Norwalk Press, 1995.

About the Author

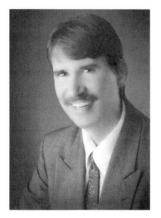

Dr. Scott C. Senne completed his Bachelor of Science at North Dakota State University, and his Doctorate in Chiropractic Medicine from Northwestern Health Sciences University. He is certified by the National Board of Chiropractic Examiners (NBCE); is a certified acupuncturist, having completed his studies at Logan College of Chiropractic; is a Certified Nutrition Specialist from the American College of Nutrition; and is certified by the American Council on Exercise as an Advanced Health and Fitness Specialist—Gold Standard. The author is also certified by the National Strength and Conditioning Association as a Strength and Conditioning Specialist. For over ten years, Dr. Senne served as administrator and practitioner to Senne Chiropractic and Acupuncture Clinic, one of the busiest healthcare practices in the Midwest, treating and advising thousands of patients. He also had privileges at North Dakota's Medcenter One Hospital.

Dr. Senne has lectured extensively on health using various media platforms, including television, radio, and print; conducts healthcare seminars throughout the United States; and has been a contributing writer for *Runner's World*, a national fitness magazine. He is the founder of Dr. Senne Health Consultant, LLC, a healthcare consulting and practice management company, and currently provides consulting services to other healthcare physicians regarding clinical, business, and practice management operations.

Dr. Senne resides in Lehigh Acres, Florida, where he is the Christian Education Director for a local church. He is married and the proud father of two children. If you have any questions or comments, feel free to contact him at www.drsenne.com.

Index